The
Immune Support
COOKBOOK

~ The ~
Immune Support
COOKBOOK

Easy, Delicious Recipes to
Support Your Health If You're
HIV Positive or Suffer From
CFIDS, Cancer, or Other
Degenerative Diseases

Mary Hale and Chris Miller

Introduction by Murray Susser, M.D.

A BIRCH LANE PRESS BOOK
Published by Carol Publishing Group

A Birch Lane Press Book
Published by Carol Publishing Group

Birch Lane Press is a registered trademark of Carol Communications, Inc.

Editorial Offices: 600 Madison Avenue, New York, N.Y. 10022
Sales and Distribution Offices: 120 Enterprise Avenue, Secaucus, N.J. 07094
In Canada: Canadian Manda Group, One Atlantic Avenue, Suite 105, Toronto, Ontario M6K 3E7
Queries regarding rights and permissions should be addressed to Carol Publishing Group, 600 Madison Avenue, New York, N.Y. 10022

Carol Publishing Group books are available at special discounts for bulk purchases, sales promotions, fund-raising, or educational purposes. Special editions can be created to specifications. For details, contact: Special Sales Department, Carol Publishing Group, 120 Enterprise Avenue, Secaucus, N.J. 07094

Manufactured in the United States of America
10 9 8 7 6 5 4 3 2 1

Library of Congress Cataloging-in-Publication Data

Hale, Mary, 1953–
    The immune support cookbook : easy, delicious recipes to support your health if you're HIV positive or suffer from CFIDS, cancer, or other degenerative diseases / Mary Hale and Chris Miller.
        p. cm.
    "A Birch Lane Press book."
    ISBN 1-55972-310-6 (hc)
    1. Nutrition. 2. Natural immunity. 3. Chronic fatigue syndrome—Diet therapy—Recipes. 4. HIV infections—Diet therapy—Recipes. 5. Cancer—Diet therapy—Recipes. 6. Degeneration (Pathology)—Nutritional aspects. I. Miller, Chris, 1942– . II. Title.
RA784.M49   1995
641.5'63—dc20   95–19245
                                                                          CIP

∽ Contents ∾

Part Three
The Phase Two Diet

Part Four
Food You Don't Prepare Yourself

Introduction
Murray Susser, M.D.

I am glad Mary and Chris have written *The Immune Support Cookbook*. It is a logical follow-up to their earlier work, *The Chronic Fatigue Syndrome Cookbook*, since CFS is but one of many forms of deficiency in the immune system.

The immune system is the body's major defense against infection and degenerative diseases like cancer. This book, therefore, helps people with chronic degenerative diseases who may not have a doctor who cares enough about nutrition to emphasize its importance or offer guidance. The recipes herein flow simply and tastefully. Equally important, they are practical—I find that even a clumsy kitchen oaf like me can negotiate them. And, once created, these nourishing and appetizing delicacies delight the palate and refresh the spirit, easing the burden disease can inflict on the basic need to eat.

Immune system weakness makes the need to eat simply and safely more imperative. It may well be that a failure to eat well is the major reason people develop weakness in the immune system. I believe the recipes here can return to the immune system victim some of the pleasure of eating that is often lost through disease. In this book, Mary and Chris make eating a joy instead of a treatment.

I have been treating Chronic Fatigue Immune Deficiency Syndrome, AIDS, and other immune system diseases for many years—in fact for about fifteen years before CFS and AIDS were given these names. Since co-writing the book *Solving the Puzzle of Chronic Fatigue Syndrome*, I have treated patients with these diseases in even greater numbers. My longstanding belief that CFS is a disease of the immune system has been reinforced again and again. My consequent belief—that the immune system can be fully treated by paying strict attention to nutrition—has also been continually reaffirmed.

The conventional treatment for AIDS does not enthrall me. It generally lacks the nutritional component that is so vital to support the immune system. Even as I write these words, studies are appearing to proclaim the importance of good nutrition to the immune system of AIDS patients. By the time this book is published, perhaps this concept will be generally accepted. Nothing would please me more. Whether or not nutrition achieves its rightful place in the conventional management of AIDS, however, this cookbook will be helpful to the AIDS patient.

Deciding upon the best diet in this complex world of modern eating is a problem that would have taxed the proverbial wisdom of Solomon. Arguments and controversy abound. No one is quite sure what the ideal diet should be for a healthy, normal human, much less for one suffering from immune deficiency. Experience, however, has taught us that the principles and techniques of this book work.

I know little about the nitty-gritty of preparing recipes, planning a meal, or shopping for ingredients. But I do know a considerable amount about reading labels, and which foods are good or bad for people with immune system problems. My role in making this book useful to immune system patients, then, is to explain how food and menu selection can support the immune and endocrine systems as patients try to maintain their health. I have been prescribing diet selection for virtually all of the fifteen thousand patients I have seen during the past twenty years.

When planning the nutritional management of patients with immune weakness, I consider many factors: sugar metabolism, weight status, digestive and bowel function, allergic status, and the function of digestive endocrines such as the pancreas and liver. I must also consider what is possible—the patient's taste, energy, resources, and willingness to accept new eating habits all add to the equation that must be solved.

When I talk about diet to my patients, the question I most often hear is "Why?" Why no sugar? Why no fruit? Why no milk? Many of the diet principles foment argument about the merits of the yeast-free diet and the low-fat diet; there is endless discussion of the pros and cons of nutritional eating. But it need not be complex; a few simple principles can make your diet measurably healthier.

Sugar, for example, is a major culprit. The average American eats about 125 pounds of the stuff in his yearly diet. That is 125 pounds too much. Sugar masquerades as food, but could rightly be called a drug with calories. It contains no nutrients—just calories. And since calories abound in the American diet while nutrients go begging, sugar may actually poison us insidiously.

That may sound like a harsh indictment of the treat we use to reward children. We know, however, that we need nutrients like vitamins B_1 and B_6 and pantothenic acid to burn sugar. Those nutrients get processed out of the sugarcane or sugar beet from which sugar comes. When the processed sugar reaches us in candy or pastry or ice cream (and in canned, packaged, and frozen foods), our bodies need to use the reserve nutrients to metabolize the sugar. If the reserve nutrients are marginal or frankly lacking, which is likely after prolonged sugar usage, we soon create a deficiency state—usually a subtle one at first. The first signs of such deficiency may be colds, flus, rash, allergy, muscle aches, etc. Emotional states like depression might follow. Next we will likely see hypogycemia (low blood sugar) and more serious immune deficiency such as pneumonia. The condition begins to resemble CFS, which acts like a flu that never gets better.

Moving on to specific foods that should be eliminated in order to insure better health and less immune dysfunction, you may wonder why processed grains are forbidden. It happens that white flour and white rice, to name two, are little more than chains of nutritionless sugars. Starches in general are chains of sugars, but the starch in the farina of a whole grain of wheat is the king in a court of juicy nutrients, most of which are destroyed. The whole wheat berry contains the germ and the bran along with the farina. When the refining of wheat removes the germ, which contains most of the vitamins, and the bran, which contains the protein and minerals, we are left with the farina—which is then bleached to kill any semblance of life that may have survived the milling. Add to the farina eight synthetic B vitamins, made from coal tar, and we get "enriched" flour. Was ever a word used more deceptively than *enriched*?

The principle now begins to take shape. Refined food, which pleases our acquired tastes, gradually robs us of our nutritional reserve. As a rule, the more primitive the food source, the more nourishment it will provide. This book recommends the use of whole wheat, unpolished rice, and all other grains in the most primitive state available. I have seen this change in diet make major differences in a person's health.

Milk restrictions will surprise many people. Milk has always enjoyed great public relations, although in recent years, it has suffered the slings of the anticholesterol campaign. But milk carries a lot of antinutritional baggage that most people do not suspect. Fat and cholesterol, by the way, are not significant evils in CFS and perhaps other immune dysfunctions. A larger problem is milk sugar. The lactose sugar in milk actually rivals the sucrose (table sugar) that permeates our pastries, ice cream, and candy. It behaves much like a processed sugar—especially in low-fat milk! The fat in whole milk acts to buffer the sugar so that it is not absorbed so quickly into the bloodstream. If one must drink milk, select whole milk (unless you have a serious cholesterol problem).

Another problem with milk is that the protein in it seems to trigger allergic reactions in many susceptible people. The allergies may be of the respiratory or skin variety, or, more insidiously, they may affect the brain, the gut, and evidently the immune system. These allergies often go unrecognized, and many orthodox medical doctors disagree as to whether they even exist. There are other problems with milk and milk products such as the addition of antibiotics and bovine growth hormone to the diets of our dairy cows. The best policy with milk products seems to be total avoidance at first and moderate, intermittent use once the problem comes under control.

That fruit may be harmful is another surprise to most people. Why avoid fruit? It comes to us fresh and raw. One of our most primitive and, therefore, desirable foods should not threaten our health. Alas, it contains a lot of sugar, and sugar can be a problem for a damaged metabolism. It changes the acidity in the gut and is absorbed quickly into the bloodstream. It peaks the blood sugar abruptly and requires many nutrients to metabolize it. It probably causes yeast to grow and metabolize more quickly, thereby increasing any toxicity that may be occurring from excess yeast growth in the gut. I tell people that fruit should be treated like exercise. Exercise is good for you unless you have a broken leg or some such injury. Fruit is good for you unless you have a broken metabolism. After you heal, you can have all you want.

Incidentally, for some people, potato behaves like fruit. The starch in potato breaks down into sugar in the mouth and hits the stomach like pure table sugar. It does not taste sweet, but it behaves sweet. Be alert. Some people can handle potato; others can't. To make things even more confusing, sweet potato is okay. It has oils in it, and does not seem to attack our sugar balance.

Food allergy plays a major role for many immune dysfunction patients. Why should anyone be allergic to food? Food allergy seems to result from a combination of two digestive errors. One: The food does not break down completely into its basic component parts. Protein, for example, should digest into individual amino acids that are easily absorbed into the bloodstream and are virtually never allergenic. Incomplete digestion of protein produces chains of amino acids called polypeptides. Polypeptides are highly allergenic, but would not cause any problem if a second digestive error did not occur, which has to do with the absorptive function of the bowel wall. If the bowel becomes damaged and dysfunctional for any reason, it may absorb these highly allergenic polypeptides. This combination of errors commonly occurs.

Alcohol and caffeine are two legal drugs that give a great deal of pleasure and have their uses. They can also do much harm when used to excess. Deciding how much is too much is difficult for a healthy person. With an immune dysfunction sufferer, the answer is usually painfully obvious: Most immune dysfunction patients cannot tolerate *any* caffeine or alcohol. Caffeine may give a temporary boost, but often delivers a devastating backlash. Similarly, alcohol can provide some temporary tranquillity, but usually hits us with an even worse backlash. Many immune dysfunction patients quickly recognize the sting of alcohol and quit drinking on their own. For many, it is more difficult to give up caffeine. But it is important to find a way to be weaned from it. When I say *weaned*, I mean it. I usually recommend decreasing by not more than 25 percent of the daily intake each week and taking three to six weeks to get off it entirely. Quitting cold turkey usually results in temporary headaches and increased fatigue. One can soften the blow by taking good vitamin supplements. That is sometimes the most important part of managing the weaning process.

I believe that nutritional supplements are a vital part of treating immune dysfunction. Many practitioners now clearly recognize the need for more vitamin and minerals than we can get from the best possible diet. I have been prescribing vitamin and mineral supplements for twenty-five years. I do so because in my experience the result has been undeniably positive. Recent medical journals have increasingly validated my experience. For decades, I have heard that my routine prescription of thirty or more vitamin pills per day is controversial at best, and many went so far as to call it quackery. Now studies from UCLA, Harvard, and other prestigious institutions are showing that supplements can cure as well as prevent disease. The purpose of this book is not to teach you about supplemental vitamins, but I would be remiss if I did not mention their importance. An excellent diet is the first order of business, but we also need supplements.

I conclude my introduction with a wish for your wellness. I believe that the principles and techniques of this cookbook will make an enormous contribution to any CFS, AIDS, or other immune dysfunction sufferer who uses it appropriately. Just remember that the raw materials of our immune system come only from food. If you use poor building materials, you will get a poor building.

Santa Monica, California

Introduction
Mary Hale

In 1984, I contracted the disease which would become known as CFIDS (Chronic Fatigue Immune Deficiency Syndrome), and my world began a slow spin into uncontrollable nightmare. I saw doctors who, while well-meaning, misdiagnosed my complaints. Since my bloodwork showed no abnormalities, many of them interpreted my exhaustion as depression. One gentle physician even hoped it *was* depression, for, as he told me, there were some disturbing new viral diseases on the horizon for which medical science, at that point, had no treatment. Indeed, he went on, these viruses could stay with one for years.

Unfortunately, he was all too right. I suffered not only the debilitating agonies of CFIDS but, because of an impaired immune system, also had to battle endrometrosis, parasites, and candida. Things got worse in 1986 when I became pregnant. I chose to go through with the pregnancy, but it was difficult. In the third trimester, I experienced pain so severe that I was confined to bed and a wheelchair, and often literally screamed in agony.

After the birth, my health slid still further. I believed I would die. Even digesting food was so exhausting I would come close to passing out after meals. My blood pressure would drop thirty points when I stood up. I could feel my heart weaken and almost stop at times. And no one could help me.

Now, on the road back to health, I look back in wonder at what I've gone through. It was an ordeal beyond my worst imaginings, yet I remind myself that there have been rewards. Though I lost a career in broadcasting I'd worked over a decade to achieve, I've gained a new, less physically demanding career as a screenwriter, and it has proved equally fulfilling. Most painfully, I've lost the ability to have more children. Yet I do have a wonderful child who, because of his experiences with my constant illness, is more sensitive than many adults. He often smiles, looks up at me, and asks, "How are you feeling today, Mommy?" Indeed, my sickness actually created a greater closeness than might otherwise have existed between me and my family—my son, Jack, and my husband, Chris.

Now, in conjunction with Chris, I have put this book together for others who suffer from degenerative, debilitating diseases. I know that changing my diet and using these recipes have helped me in regaining my health, a process that is ongoing. Though I'm not yet where I want to be, I've come a million miles from where I started, and continue to get better day by day.

Before signing off, I want to stress the point Dr. Susser made in his introduction: the recipes in this book *will* make a difference for you. They will support your immune system, which will help you feel better, think clearer, and lead a happier life. And they will return to you something you may have thought your new dietary requirements would permanently deprive you of—the pleasure of eating not simply healthy, but healthy *and* delicious food.

Enjoy.

Introduction
Chris Miller

For me, eating is about pleasure. The three most important events of my day are breakfast, lunch, and dinner. I *love* food.

Over the years, I realized that if I *really* wanted to eat well, I'd have to learn how to cook for myself—what I could get at restaurants too often disappointed me. So I became a pretty fair chef. I learned how to whip up French sauces, Italian pastas, sweet Thai concoctions, Japanese sushi, and American cheese-burgers, cookies, and cakes.

Imagine my horror when I found out my wife—the woman I plan to spend the rest of my life with—had contracted some weird disease that would allow her to eat none of the above! In fact, her list of forbidden foods looked nine miles long, while what she *could* eat seemed restricted to rice cakes, nut butter, and air.

I felt bad for her, but also for myself. How was I going to survive on this diet she had to follow so scrupulously? Was my greatest pleasure to be taken from me?

But no. What I discovered was that a perfectly delicious menu of foods was still very much achievable, despite the necessity of staying within the parameters of The Diet. It took time and was sometimes frustrating, but I was able to assemble a large number of tasty, healthy recipes—which we now pass on to you.

Ironically, I wound up preferring this diet to my old one, with its rich sauces and so forth. I feel better, look better, lost weight, and have fewer worries about cholesterol and today's other nutritional bugaboos. So, in my dogged pursuit of hedonistic dining despite Mary's health problems, I actually wound up improving my own physical and emotional well-being!

And as for *you*, this book will make it possible to eat well, despite your health problems. *Bon appétit!*

PART ONE

Getting Oriented

∽ 1 ∾

Diet and Disease

You're sick. You feel awful. The pain can be overwhelming. Normal people have no concept of what you're going through, and the anxiety of making it through each day with no relief in sight is making you sicker.

Although doctors, OMDs (doctors of oriental medicine), acupuncturists, and other health care providers often differ on how to treat chronic illnesses, one thing they almost all agree on is that a special diet is essential to getting better.

The healthy diet should:

a) Avoid all substances that are generally held to be unhealthy: sugar, alcohol, fried foods, etc. The conventional wisdom about these edibles is true—they're bad for you.

b) Eliminate all substances to which you are allergic. Many people with an autoimmune disease also suffer from allergies—there's a high correspondence between the two. Your physician can help determine what your allergies are. *You will particularly need to determine whether you have contracted a systemic yeast infection known as candida. If you have, you will be susceptible to a number of cross-allergies that could rule out consuming baker's yeast, mushrooms, vinegar, and other foods.*

The recipes in this cookbook adhere to these rules. We realize that health care professionals will differ on what foods should and should not be allowed in your diet. That's why the ingredients we use here are conservative, and should do you no harm, no matter what particular degenerative disease you're suffering from.

3

The Bad News and the Good News

No way around it, you're faced with a double whammy. Not only is a chronic disease making you miserable, now there's this stringent new diet you have to follow. The list of things you're not allowed to eat is long, and certain to contain at least three dozen items you can't live without. And when you see the list of what you *can* eat, you'll wonder "How can I possibly survive on this?"

When you're so tired and sick that brushing your teeth can seem like running a marathon, the job of revamping the entire way you eat seems impossible. Foods you've taken for granted all your life are suddenly verboten: the frozen dinners you popped in the microwave on nights you got home late contain sugar and other taboo ingredients; the wine you liked with lamb chops is mainly distilled sugar; you can't eat pizza (cheese), or takeout Chinese (MSG, soy sauce), or one single thing at McDonald's (sugar, cheese, God knows what else).

The world, you quickly discover, is not set up for people with a degenerative disease.

But here's the good news: With a little thought and planning, and the help of this book, creating new eating habits isn't nearly the insurmountable task you think it is. *Not only can you eat healthily, you can eat well.*

The recipes contained herein are as normal as scrambled eggs, green salads, and pasta. It's bad enough you don't feel well—you don't need to endure a "health food" (to many people, a code word for "bland" or "weird") diet as well. Your authors are mainstream food lovers, not self-denying health obsessives trying to force you to live on beansprouts and tofu. The recipes in this book have been composed to appeal to any lover of food and eating.

Your Diet's Two Phases

Most doctors and health care professionals who treat chronic illness ask their patients to radically change their diet. As we have already discussed, good nutrition is vital to maintaining health; that's why we have created two phases for this chronic disease diet.

Phase One is really a clean-out diet. People have unique reactions to foods. What's good for one may not be good for another. Each of you will have to discover which foods work for you. We recommend, as do many nutritionists, that you keep a food diary in which you record each day what you eat, and what reactions, if any, occur. By "reactions," we refer to bloating, gas, muscle pain, depression, fatigue, itching, etc. Phase One should clean out your system, so that when you reintroduce foods, you can gauge your reaction to them.

Most important in Phase One is to eliminate preservatives, sugar, caffeine, and allergy-causing foods from your body. As you do this, your immune system will become stronger and you should feel better. Eating "bad" foods only makes you sicker—and you certainly don't need that.

For this reason, the Phase One diet is the more restrictive one. Most of the recipes in this book are for Phase One. (Don't worry, they still taste great.) Once you've regained a certain degree of wellness, experiencing more good days than bad and an increased energy throughout most of the day, you can try reintroducing foods such as fruit and wheat to see if you are allergic to them, or if you are strong enough now to tolerate them.

There are, by the way, blood tests that can tell you what you are allergic to. They are fine, but simple trial and error is also helpful. Listen to your body. Even after years of improved health, sugar may still cause muscle aches, so try to avoid it, as well as all alcohol and caffeine. Phase One is by and large the way we prefer to eat almost every day.

A word of warning: In the beginning, the cleansing process makes some people feel worse. But as the diet "kicks in," you will experience a return of mental clarity and physical energy you'd almost forgotten you could feel. It's then you'll discover what this diet can truly mean for you.

When you move to Phase Two, this does not mean you should give up the recipes in Phase One, which you can enjoy for the rest of your life, if you wish. Many of them can easily be "upgraded" to become part of the less-restrictive Phase Two diet. In the case of pasta, for instance, merely substitute wheat pasta (assuming you have not discovered you are allergic to wheat) for wheatless.

Here's the list of what you can and can't eat. Make a copy and take it shopping with you. Don't worry, you'll soon have it memorized. And remember—*always read ingredient lists.*

Forbidden Foods

1. *Sugar*   A.k.a. sucrose, glucose, fruit sugar, dextrose, dextrins, dextran, diastase, diastatic malt, ethyl maltol, sorbitol, corn sweeteners, caramel, carob syrup, fructose, high-fructose corn syrup, honey, molasses, brown sugar, fruit juice, maple syrup, brown rice syrup, steria, etc. This also includes artificial sweeteners—Nutrasweet, Sweet 'N Low, and the like. Sugar is the *number-one* item you must avoid. *If you do nothing else, eliminate sugar from your diet.*

2. *Milk Products*   Milk, cream, cheese, yogurt, sour cream, ice cream, etc. The reasons for this are simple: Milk products contain sugar, and many people are allergic to them. There is ample evidence that the increased use of antibiotics and bovine growth hormone in our dairy cattle may cause toxic reactions and harm the immune system.

3. *Yeast-Containing Foods* *If* you're allergic to them. That means tofu and miso. Also anything fermented—beer, wine, sake, champagne, soy sauce, vinegar. Also most breads, rolls, cakes, and so forth; yeast is what makes most of them rise.

4. *Alcohol* It's best to stay away from alcohol completely, but when you don't, drink tequila or vodka, and do so in moderation.

5. *Mushrooms* If you have an allergy to mushrooms or yeast, watch out. Fungi are mold, as is yeast. If you're not allergic, you can eat mushrooms whenever you like— especially the shiitake mushroom. This wonderful-tasting delicacy may even have immune-stimulating characteristics.

6. *Fruits* Fruits are too sweet, and many contain yeast and ferment easily. Fruit juice, even freshly squeezed, is also forbidden. However, when you reach Phase Two of your diet, try reintroducing fruits, one at a time, to see if you can tolerate them.

7. *Tea and Coffee* This includes decaffeinated tea and coffee. Herb teas are okay, however. Especially pau d'arco, which you can find at a health food store. This tea from South America may actually kill yeast.

8. *Commercial Mustards and Mayonnaise* Many store-bought mustards and mayonnaise contain vinegar, a definite no-no for the chronically ill patients who are allergic to the yeast in it. Try making your own mayonnaise (our recipe is on page 157) or if you don't want to chance salmonella poisoning from raw eggs, try a health-food brand.

9. *Fried Foods*

10. *Wheat and Rye* Again, only if you're allergic. Of course, most crackers, cereals, pastas, breads, etc. are made from wheat flour. If you don't have an allergy to wheat, however, don't deny yourself.

11. *Ketchups, Tomato Sauces, Barbecue Sauces* Not unless you make your own—without vinegar, syrup, or sugar.

12. *Miscellaneous No-Nos* Horseradish. Oatmeal. Potatoes.

Allowed Foods

1. *Poultry* Chicken, duck, goose, pheasant, turkey, chicken liver, and liver pâté.

2. *Most Fish* Abalone, bass, bluefish, carp, catfish, caviar, clam, crab, cod, eel, flounder, haddock, halibut, herring, lobster, mackerel,* oyster, perch, pike, pollock, salmon (fresh*), oyster, sardines, scallops, shad,* shrimp, smelt, snails, snapper, swordfish,** trout,* tuna,** wakeme, whitefish.*

3. *All Vegetables and Fresh Vegetable Juices*

4. *Selected Fruits and Fresh-Squeezed Fruit Juices* Proceed with caution. As mentioned, fruit contains a lot of natural sugar, and a weakened immune system may not tolerate it. But if eating fruit causes you no major problems, try papaya, mango, kiwi, pineapple, banana, honeydew melon, coconut, guava, lemons, and limes. Also the juices of these, and unsweetened cranberry juice. Best to eat these fruits only in the morning.

6. *Grains and Beans* Whole, unprocessed brown rice, wild rice, millet, buckwheat, quinoa, and amaranth. Avoid white rice. It's a good idea to combine grains and beans to make a complete protein.

---

*high fat
**high mercury

7. *Margarine and Eggs*   Look for margarine with "Made Without Animal Products" on the label.

8. *Nuts*   Except peanuts and pistachios, which harbor mold.

9. *Rice Cakes, Rice Crackers (made from whole unprocessed rice), Corn Tortillas, Corn Chips, Popcorn*

10. *Rice Noodles, Japanese Buckwheat Noodles (Goba), Quinoa Pasta, Corn Pasta, Amaranth Pasta*

11. *Meat*   Lamb, veal, rabbit. Limit to no more than two servings per week, due to fat and difficulty in digesting. Avoid processed meats such as sausage, ham, and bacon.

A Note About Salt

We haven't included salt in our recipes, instead leaving the decision to use or not to use up to you. Dr. Susser believes that only if you have heart trouble, hypertension, or problems with water retention do you need to worry about salt. In fact, he says, many who pursue health and fitness make the mistake of cutting *too* much salt out of their diet. Salt, in moderation, is good.

Many food flavors can be greatly improved by the judicious use of salt. So feel free to add some as you cook, or sprinkle some at the table. You will notice that some of our recipes call for unsalted butter or margarine. That's merely because the outcome tastes better that way. Our number-one priority, after feeding you nothing that can hurt you, is feeding you meals that are delicious and can reintroduce sensual pleasure to your life, despite your illness.

A Note About Butter

In our opinion, no substitute tastes as good as butter. But the dairy industry's use of antibiotics and bovine growth hormone may be reason enough to avoid the real thing. If you feel, as we do, that your food should be as pure and wholesome as possible, try substituting safflower oil. Or find one that states on the label "no animal products" (many margarines have whey—a milk protein).

However, as with salt, a bit of butter here and there isn't going to kill you. If you feel comfortable using butter in moderation, by all means do so. This is why you will often see the words "margarine or butter" in our recipes. It's really your call.

SUBSTITUTIONS

When a recipe calls for an ingredient that you can't tolerate, maybe you can find a substitute. Here's a by-no-means exhaustive list of substitutions that have worked for us.

Recipe Calls For:	*Instead Use:*
Milk	Dairy substitutes, usually rice- or soy-derived
Cheese	Soy cheese
Vinegar	Lemon juice
Mayonnaise	Homemade (see chapter 8) or health food substitute
Flour (wheat)	Amaranth, barley, brown rice, buckwheat, millet, oat, quinoa, rice, and soy flours
White wine	Chicken broth

Bread	Tortillas or other unleavened bread (corn tortillas, if you can't have wheat), ponce bread, and rice bread
Pasta	Rice noodles, Japanese buckwheat noodles, quinoa pasta, corn pasta, amaranth pasta

A Coping Strategy

There will be times when you'll be too tired even to *think* about cooking. That's when you go to the freezer for a meal you've cooked previously. Or throw together the ultra-easy, ultra-quick foods described in the chapter after next, Mary's Quickies.

The number-one rule is: *Avoid bad ingredients.* But this is a rule that can and probably should be broken once in a while. The number-two (and equally important) rule is: *Be good to yourself.* We recommend adhering to a formula suggested by Dr. Susser—a 19:2 Ratio—if nineteen of your twenty-one weekly meals are dietetically correct, give yourself a break on the other two. Yield to temptation and go for that slice of pepperoni pizza you've been mentally salivating over—you may even find that as times goes by, you're not missing these foods as much as you once did.

Though alcoholic beverages are inescapably on your forbidden list, even here you can give yourself the occasional treat. Vodka's safest. Stolichnaya, Absolut, or Icy are tasty and eye-opening. Try them on the rocks with a squeeze of lemon or lime or straight from the freezer—which renders them thick and oily—with buffalo grass or a grind of pepper.

Having a chronic illness doesn't mean you must retire from the human race. The occasional forbidden pleasure reaffirms your humanness. Just don't make a habit of it.

Meanwhile, give yourself as many *allowed* pleasures as possible: hot tubs, massages, beautiful sunsets, and cut flowers. Managing your disease makes you enough of a self-denier by itself—compensate by developing an indulgent, generous relationship with yourself in other areas.

Stress, as has been widely published, is one of the biggest blocks to maintaining good health. You must counterbalance its destructiveness. Unfortunately this is difficult. Fatigue and depression can easily lead to a horrible cycle of bad eating habits, nonexercising, and total couch-potatohood. So be good to yourself. Ask your family and friends to help by taking you to the movies or for a walk, or just to sit peacefully with you and read a book. Loving care and compassion are some of the best medicines on your road to feeling as good as you can.

～ 2 ～

Equipment

B ecause you're often tired, whatever makes life easier is good. Nonstick pots and pans, for instance. Electric can openers are also good. Wherever possible, simplify.

Freezer

You'll learn to exploit your freezer like never before. On nights you don't feel like cooking, pull something out that you cooked previously and froze in one- or two-person quantities. Get lots of those little plastic freezer containers and bags from the supermarket, and keep an inventory of selections at all times.

Microwave Ovens

A microwave is a big help. It can reheat your pau d'arco tea, cook vegetables and fish to perfection, warm your plates, boil water, and resuscitate your dinner after interruptions by children or phones. We use one constantly.

We probably should not neglect to mention, however, that microwaves emit low-level electromagnetic waves. Studies have linked these to birth defects, miscarriage, and various forms of cancer. Though we don't let this cheery news bother us—and use the 'wave constantly anyway—we want you to have all the information you need to make your own decision.

Steamers

Steamers provide another great, healthy way to cook vegetables. Get one of the metal, fold-open ones. It won't cost much, and you'll use it a lot.

Grill

Using an indoor grill on your cooktop is a great way to cook entire dinners that are healthy and easy. Outdoor grills are also fine—even a small hibachi will do the trick.

Juicer

One of your tickets to continued health is freshly juiced vegetables, which, as a bonus, turn out to be delicious. If you don't have a juice bar situated around the corner, you might want to invest in a juicer. Fresh vegetable juices are also available in many health food stores (see chapter 3).

Wok

Inexpensive and endlessly useful. Stir-fried food is fast, easy, healthy, delicious, and fun. Those leftovers you have in the refrigerator can be thrown into the wok with a little oil and rice and *voilà*—instant lunch or dinner. You can wrap your creation in a warmed tortilla. Also good for making soups, eggs, sauces—almost anything.

Miscellaneous

Of course, you'll need all the equipment any other cook needs—wooden spoons, a meat thermometer, a timer that goes *ping* when your food's ready. Food processors are very helpful—the time and aggravation they save make them worth the price. A Mouli grater works best for our grating needs.

Again, anything that makes life easier is good. A trash container with a foot pedal is better than one you have to open by hand. A sprayer attachment on your sink makes cleaning dishes a snap. Chopping boards keep the counters clean. Dust Busters are great for dealing with dry spills. You get the idea.

In this spirit, please feel free to take as many shortcuts with these recipes as you like. Instead of peeling and seeding tomatoes, buy already peeled and seeded tomatoes in a can. If you don't have a particular ingredient on hand, be adventurous and substitute. Ask your butcher to cut and slice fish, poultry, and meat, so you don't have to. Take the shortcuts and just enjoy the nutritious, balanced diet this book can give you.

⏤ 3 ⏤

Shopping

Shopping's a whole new ball game when there's an immune deficiency disease in your family. As with cooking and eating, you have to revamp your methodology. This may seem daunting at first. The extra label-reading is an annoyance. But, as with the other changes disease forces on your life, you quickly incorporate it and it becomes second nature.

Ingredient Lists

From now on, buy nothing until you've read the label. You won't *believe* the places sugar turns up. It's in bread and bacon, frozen french fries and tomato soup. It's in toothpaste and most chicken broths. It's even in many pain relievers.

There's milk in soda crackers and canned soups, yeast in sauerkraut and canned tomato sauce, wheat in liverwurst and bouillon cubes. It's a minefield out there.

What are you supposed to do? Read the ingredient lists. When you're buying ready-to-eat foods, *ask* what the ingredients are. More often than not your suspicions will be justified.

By and large, you'll do better at health food stores than commercial supermarkets. You're more likely to find the products you're looking for—without sugar, refined flour, or caffeine. But even here you have to look out for the miso and honey. You must be endlessly vigilant.

You may wonder if there are any foods that are *not* contaminated. As far as packaged, canned, and frozen foods are concerned—very few. Whenever possible, use fresh ingredients and make your own food. When not possible, read labels carefully.

What label ingredients should you seek to avoid? Here's a list. It's by no means exhaustive, but it covers the main areas. Copy and take it along while shopping until you've learned it.

COMMON FORBIDDEN INGREDIENTS

Aspartame
Beet juice concentrate
Corn syrup
Dextrose
Fructose
High-fructose corn syrup
Hydrolyzed protein

Modified food
    starch
Potassium sorbate
Pyrophosphate
Sucrose
Sugar syrup
Yeast extract*

COMMON FOODS TO AVOID

Barbecue sauce
Beer
Bread*
Cakes
Cheese
Cookies
Cream
Crackers
Enriched flours
Mayonnaise
Milk

Olives
Pastries
Pickles
Pretzels
Rolls
Salad dressings
Sauerkraut
Soy sauce
Vinegar*
Wine

---

*Avoid these items only if you're allergic to them. The rule of thumb is: When in doubt, avoid them. We have, therefore, included no recipes containing these possible allergens in the Phase One section of this book.

Chicken Broth

One ingredient we'll call for again and again is chicken broth. There's a fairly easy recipe for chicken stock in chapter 8. But if you're like us, you won't find time to make it very often. Often you'll need to use the canned chicken broth.

And when you do, you'll experience the ingredient problem in microcosm. Though there are many commercial chicken broths, most of them contain sugar! Two that we've found do not—Pritikin and Jewish Mother brands. Maybe you can discover others.

Going to Market

Shopping at the supermarket is an ordeal. It sometimes seems impossible to stand in the aisle reading labels on endless packages while suffering every conceivable pain. Even parenting isn't as exhausting as grocery shopping. But when you don't have the energy to cook, you need to have something in the house that you can just heat up. Following are some ready-to-eat foods that for the most part fit the diet or have only one questionable ingredient.

Again, this is not an exhaustive list, but it should help you identify the items that are the least harmful and are in some rare cases actually good for you. The list is in two parts: foods generally found in your standard supermarket and those found in health food stores. It should come as no surprise where you'll have more choices.

Since most of the brands listed below in the standard supermarket section are national brands, you shouldn't have any trouble locating them no matter where you live in the United States.

SUPERMARKETS

Snack Foods:

Amsnack Gourmet Rice Snax
Bell Natural Style Corn Chips (salt)
Chico San Sesame Rice Cakes or Popcorn Cakes
Hain Mini Popcorn Rice Cakes (salt)
Hain Butter-Flavored Popcorn (salt)
Eagle Lightly Salted Tortilla Chips (salt)
Jiffy Pop Natural Flavor Popcorn (salt)
Weight Watchers Popcorn (salt)

Salsas and Sauces:

El Paso Salsa de Jalapeño (salt)
Herdez Salsa Casera, mild, medium, and hot (salt)
Herdez Salsa Verde (salt)
Ortega Green Chile Salsa (salt)
Ortega Dried Jalapeños (salt)
Rosarita Enchilada Sauce (salt)

Cereals:

El Molino Puffed Corn
Kolln Oat Bran Crunch (barley malt)
Malt-O-Meal Puffed Rice
Mother's Oat Bran
Nabisco Cream of Rice
Quaker Oat Bran—look for the "no salt, no sugar" on
   the package

Soups:

Andersen's Split Pea Soup (salt)
Hain Vegetable Chicken Soup

Health Valley Fat-Free Soups:
  Vegetable Barley
  Real Italian Minestrone (whole-wheat macaroni)
  14 Garden Vegetable
  Country Corn & Vegetable
  Chicken Broth (grape juice)
  Manhattan Clam Chowder (soy oil)
  5 Bean Vegetable
Jewish Mother Chicken Broth
Jewish Mother Chicken Vegetable Soup (salt)
Jewish Mother Chicken Vegetable Rice (salt)
Pritikin Chicken Broth
Pritikin Split Pea Soup (salt)
Pritikin Minestrone Soup (cooked macaroni product)

Most of these soups will be found in the health food section of the supermarket. This varies by store, however, and in many smaller markets you may not find them at all.

Canned Vegetables:

  Green Giant Golden Sweet Corn—look for the "no salt or sugar added" on the package
  Hunt's Whole Tomatoes (salt)
  Progresso Crushed Tomatoes (salt)

It's very difficut to find any canned vegetable in regular supermarkets that isn't made with sugar—read labels.

Frozen Vegetables:

You'll have much better luck with frozen vegetables than with canned.

C & W frozen vegetables state right on the package that nothing is added; the only exception might be salt. The same goes for Birds Eye and Green Giant frozen vegetables. All three manufacturers freeze only the vegetables, occasionally with a trace of salt.

Tomato Pasta Sauces:
Contadina's Fresh Marinara Sauce (salt)
Enrico's Spaghetti Sauce
Enrico's Pasta Sauce
Romance's Fresh Marinara Sauce (salt)
Weight Watchers Spaghetti Sauce Flavored With Meat

Rice and Grains:
Pritikin Spanish Brown Rice

Frozen Soups:
Tabatchnik Soups
   Barley Bean
   Pea—look for the "no salt—no sugar added"
   Northern Bean

Unfortunately, virtually all frozen meals (Lean Cuisine, Weight Watchers, Swanson's, etc.) make dishes with cream sauces, wheat pasta, and other forbidden ingredients. You have no choice but to stay away from them, even though using them would make life a whole lot simpler.

If you're lucky enough to have a supermarket that has a "Special" or "Foreign" foods section, inspect it closely. Many of the items there will be good for your restrictive diet. For instance, try substituting Chinese rice noodles or bean threads for pasta. In the Mexican cuisine arena, there are a multitude of beans and salsas that might work, and Middle Eastern delicacies such as tahini, sesame butter, and eggplant dip are delicious and most are free of bad ingredients.

One final note: Anyone suffering from a chronic disease needs pain relievers. Here, too, you must read labels carefully. Regular and Extra-Strength Tylenol are good, but the gel caps contain dyes. Excedrin Extra Strength contains sixty-five milligrams of caffeine per tablet. The shell around Advil contains sucrose, and Nuprin products contain dyes. You may have to choose between the least of many evils.

HEALTH FOOD STORES

You'll have a higher shopping batting average in health food stores. Products there tend to be more expensive, but you'll find a larger variety of acceptable foods. The fruits and vegetables offered are more likely to be organically grown and pesticide-free.

Following is a list of foods that we find especially helpful. Once again, this is not an all-inclusive list, but it will get you started.

Even though health food store products are generally better, you must still be vigilant. Some manufacturers' products will work for you and others won't.

In health food stores, some of the brands are regional, meaning that what may be readily available to us in Southern California may not make its way to the upper expanses of Maine. Look for your own regional brands for some different and refreshing taste treats.

However, the consumer demand for good food in the last decade has resulted in a dizzying array of delicious, nutritious national products. Many are listed here.

For your convenience we have marked the national brands with an *N* and the regional brands (our region being Southern California) with an *R*.

Ready-made Salads:

Spa Salads (R)
  Broccoli Corn Bean
  Brown Rice Sauté
  Daily Greens with
    Lemon Pesto

Garlic Brown Rice
Steamed Brown Rice
Steamed Brown Rice and
  Vegetables
Seven Grain

Freshly Squeezed Juices (fruit juices for Phase Two diet only):

Amazake (N)
  Almond Shake
  Mocha-Java
  Original Flavor Shake
  Vanilla Pecan Shake
Chiquita (N)
  Papaya Smoothie
  Protein Pump
Ferraro's Juices (R)
  Fresh Garden
    Vegetable
  Green Mix
  Lime
  Papaya Coconut
    Cremè
  Pineapple Coconut
  Pineapple Mango
  Pineapple Papaya
  Protein Colada

Salad in a Bottle
Tropical Treat
Veg-O-Green
Veg-O-Mato
Hansen's (R)
  Coconut Juice
  Protein Pick-Up
Mighty Soy (R)
  Original
Naked Foods Juices (R)
  Carrot, Parsley, &
    Spinach
  Papaya & Pineapple
  Organic Carrot
  Carrot & Beet
Rice Dream (N)
  Organic Original
  Vanilla Lite

Milk Substitutes:

Rice
  Almond Mylk
    Original
    Vanilla
  Rice Dream
    Chocolate
    Original
    Carob
    Vanilla
  Edensoy
    Original
    Carob
    Vanilla
    Extra
  Vita Soy
    Creamy Original

Vanilla
Vanilla Delite
Carob Supreme
Original
West Soy
  Vanilla
  Plain
  Original
  Cocoa
Soy Moo
Mighty Soy (R)
  Vanilla
  Carob
  Original
Amazake (N)
  Almond

Cheese Substitutes:

Silken Tofu
  Soft
  Firm
  Extra Firm
San Diego Soy
  Dairy Tofu
Super Firm Tofu
Organic Tofu
Mori-Nu Tofu

Tofu Rella
  Cheddar
  Mozzarella
Soy Gourmet
  Cheddar Style
Almond Cheeze
  Cheddar Style
Nu Tofu
  Mozzarella Flavor

Soya Kaas
  Mozzarella Style
  Mild American
    Cheddar Style
  Jalapeño Mexi-Kass
  Mild American Style
  Jalapeño Monterrey
    Jack Style

Cheddar Flavor
Monterrey Jack Flavor
Soya Melt
  Cheddar Flavor
  Mozzarella Flavor

Ice Cream Substitutes*:
Rice Dream (N)
  Carob Chip
  Cappuccino
  Vanilla
  Chocolate Marble
    Fudge
  Peanut Butter Fudge
  Vanilla Swiss Almond
  Lemon
  Carob Almond
  Wild Berry
  Vanilla Fudge
  Mint Carob Chip

Vanilla
Carob Peppermint
Almond Pecan
Raspberry
Chocolate
Chocolate Almond
Mint Carob Chip
Vanilla Swiss Almond
Sweet Nothings
  Vanilla Fudge
  Vanilla
  Chocolate Mandarin
  Verry Berry

---

*All these sweet desserts use either brown rice syrup, a fruit concentrate, or both to make them sweet. Your body may not be ready to handle all this sweetness, but when it is, better these dairy and sugar alternatives than the real thing.

Ice Cream Substitutes (continued):

Cocoa Marble Fudge
Cookie & Dream
Living Lightly
  Chocolate Almond
  Peanut Butter Cup
  Expresso

Espresso
Black Leopard
Chocolate
Mango Raspberry

Salsas and Dips:

Scotty's (R)
  Cajun Style
    Guacamole (salt)
  Fresh Salsa, Chunky
    Style (salt)
  Fresh Salsa, Herbs
    & Spices (salt)

Fresh Salsa,
  Tomatillos (salt)
Senor Felix's (R)
Salsa, Mild
Salsa, Medium Hot

Chips:

Blue Corn (N)
  Bearitos
Barbara's (N)
  Pinta Chips
Garden of Eatin' (N)
  Blue Chips—look
    for the "no salt
    added"
  Sesame Blues

Sunny Blues
  Yankee Doodles
Lapidus (N)
  Lite Corn—look for
    the "oil-free"
Popcorn
Skinny (N)
  Natural Corn Chips—
    look for the "no salt"

Bottled Juices:

Hienke's (N)
  100 Percent Cranberry
    Juice—look
    for the
    "unsweetened"

L & A
  Pineapple Coconut

Frozen Vegetables:

Cascadian Farm (N)
  Broccoli Cuts
  Corn
  Cut Green Beans
  French Fries
  Gardener's Blend
  Petits Pois (trace of salt)
  Sliced Carrots
C & W (N)
  Chopped Spinach
  French Cut Beans

  Petite Peas—look for the "no salt added"
  Petite Sweet Corn— look for the "sodium free"
  Whole Baby Carrots
  Whole Italian Green Beans
Health Valley (N)
  Leaf Spinach
  Whole Kernel Corn

Frozen Foods:

Amy's (N)
  Mexican Tamale Pies
Dos Banderos (R)
  Chicken Tamales
Jacyln's (N)
  Split Pea Soup
Mudpie (N)
  Veggie Burgers
Natural Touch (N)
  Lentil Rice Loaf

Tai (N)
  Channa Masala: chickpeas
  Raj Mah: kidney beans
Tumaro's (N)
  Black Bean Enchiladas
  Two-Bean Tamales

Pasta:

Ancient Harvest (N)
  Quinoa Pasta
Cleopatra Amaranth
  Pasta (N)
  Kamut Pasta
De Boles (N)
  Corn Pasta Elbows
  Corn Pasta
    Spaghetti
Mrs. Leeper's (N)
  Rice Pasta
Orgran (N)

Barley & Spinach
  Pasta
  Corn Pasta
Pastariso (N)
  100 Percent Rice Pasta
    Elbows
  100 Percent Rice Pasta
    Spaghetti Style
Vita-Spelt (N)
  Whole Spelt Pasta
Buonapasta (R)
  Fresh Marinara Sauce

Tomato Sauces:

Enrico's (N)
  Traditional Sauce
Hagerty Foods (N)
  Artichoke Pasta
    Sauce

Mama Cocco's (N)
  Marinara Sauce

Dehydrated Soups:

Taste Adventure (N)
  Black Bean Chili
  Curry Lentil
  Lentil Chili
  Red Bean Chili

  Split Pea Soup
The Spice Hunter (N)
  Brown & Wild
    Rice Almondine

Canned Soups:
  Hain (N)
    Turkey Rice Soup
    Vegetarian Chicken
      Broth (salt)
    Vegetarian Chicken
      Soup (salt)
    99 Percent Fat-Free
      Vegetarian Split
      Pea Soup
    99 Percent Fat-Free
      Vegetarian
      Lentil Soup
  Health Valley (N)
    5 Bean Vegetable
      Soup
    Manhattan Clam
      Chowder

  Pritikin (N)
    Chicken Broth
    Chicken Gumbo
    Lentil Soup
    Navy Bean Soup
    Split Pea Soup
  Shelton's
    Black Bean &
      Chicken Soup
    Chicken Broth
    Chicken Chili
    Turkey Chili
    Turkey Rice Soup
    Vegetable Chicken
      Soup

Grain Dishes*:
  Ancient Harvest (N)
    Quinoa
  Arrowhead Mills (N)
    Blue Cornmeal
    Quick Brown Rice
    Whole Grain Teff

  Jerusalem Falafal
    Vegetable Burger
      Mix
  Lundberg (N)
    Rizcous

---

*You will find a wonderful variety of nonwheat flours in many health food stores. Experiment and discover what best suits your taste. We personally enjoy the rice flours, but why limit yourself when you can try any or all of the following: soy flour, oat flour, cornmeal, brown rice flour, buckwheat flour, millet flour, teff flour, and amaranth flour?

Cereals:

Arrowhead Mills (N)
  Barley Flakes
  Bits O Barley
  Nature Puffs
  Nature O's
  Oat Bran
  Puffed Corn
  Puffed Millet
  Puffed Rice
Bob's Red Mill (N)
  8 Grain Wheatless
    Hot Cereal
Breadshop (N)
  Triple Bran

Ener G (N)
  Pure Rice Bran
Erewhon (N)
  Brown Rice Cream
  Oat Bran
Lundberg (N)
  Creamy Rice
Pocono (N)
  Cream of Buckwheat
Quick 'n Creamy (N)
  Brown Rice Hot
    Cereal
Tattorie Pandea
  Instant Polenta

Snacks and Miscellaneous:

Cedarlane (R)
  Eggplant Caviar
  Hummus
  Potato Salad
Edward & Sons (N)
  Onion-Garlic Brown
    Rice Snaps
  Sesame Baked
    Brown Rice Snaps

Organic Rice Cakes
Organic Rice Cakes—
  Brown Rice
Organic Rice Cakes—
  Mochi Sweet
Organic Rice Cakes—
  Popcorn
Organic Rice Cakes—
  Wild Rice

Hol-Grain (N)
  Brown Rice Lite
  Snack Thins
Judith's Natural Deli (R)
  Hummus
Lundberg (N)
  Organic Brown Rice
  Mini Rice Cakes

Premier Japan (N)
  No Salt Sesame Rice
  Sembei Crackers
Pritikin (N)
  Rice Cakes—
  Multigrain
  Rice Cakes—Sesame

***Butters**:**
Hain (N)
  Almond Butter
Roaster Fresh
  Almond Butter
  Cashew Butter
  Sunflower Butter

Westbrae Natural (N)
  Raw Cashew Butter
  Roasted Cashew
  Butter
  Smooth Almond
  Butter

---

*These butters spread on a rice cake with margarine or butter make a great instant snack.

PART TWO

The Phase One Diet

❧ 4 ❧

Mary's Quickies

On your worst days, when you can't imagine cooking or shopping, have this stuff around to get you through the day.

Popcorn

Healthy, tasty, and on-target for your diet. And easy—get the microwave kind, if you have a microwave, or the stovetop kind if you don't. Check ingredient lists to be sure the manufacturer hasn't put in forbidden ingredients such as cheese.

Nuts

Other than peanuts and pistachios, you can eat all nuts. Have you savored a roasted cashew lately? Nuts can become your candy substitute. Unfortunately, like candy, nuts pack a lot of calories, so keep that in mind. They can also be hard to digest. Enjoy them, but don't live on them.

Nut Butter on Rice Cakes

Again with the exception of butters made from peanuts or pistachios, nut butters are on the okay list. They're delicious on rice cakes. Top off with sliced bananas, if you're eating fruit, or if you're not, a layer of "good" mayonnaise.

❧

WARMING "TEA"

1 cup hot water
1/4 teaspoon of concentrated Vitamin C powder (found in
 health food stores), a squeeze of lemon or lime, or add a
 dry parsley leaf—it cleanses the bladder.

Mix in a mug. This is nice in the morning, or before bed.

❧

QUICKIE SALAD

2 fresh tomatoes, sliced   Extra-virgin olive oil
Fresh basil leaves   1/2 teaspoon lemon juice

On serving plates, alternate slices of tomatoes and basil leaves
around the outside of the plate until a semicircle is formed.
Drizzle with olive oil and lemon juice. Serve.

2 servings

🐟

QUICK STIR-FRY

This fast meal is all about exploiting whatever you have available. Stir-fry rice, vegetables, and whatever unfinished frozen dinner portions are kicking around your freezer. If you're using tomatoes, add them last and cook for only 30 seconds, so they don't fall apart. Eat wrapped up in tortillas, or on a plate.

1 tablespoon vegetable oil
Cooked rice

Leftovers — whatever's in the vegetable tray or freezer

Heat oil in a wok or medium-size skillet. Add rice and all other ingredients. Cook for 3 to 4 minutes, stirring constantly, until all vegetables are tender. A little bit of sesame oil and lemon juice add nice flavor notes to this simple meal.

Possible ingredients:
Onion
Tomatoes
Tuna, packed in water or oil
Celery
Broccoli
Dry-roasted nuts
Leftover fish, chicken, or meat

৩ 5 ৩

Breakfast

People usually think of breakfast dishes as cereal, pancakes, and sausage, bacon, and eggs. Thinking like this will drive you crazy if you're attempting to follow a healthier diet: Milk is not allowed, maple syrup is even more not allowed, and most store-brand sausage is full of chemicals and sugar. Bacon is out—like sausage, it's usually made with sugar. Still, everybody needs a good, filling start to the day. So be adventurous and stray from the beaten path. A pasta or rice dish can be a wonderful, sustaining substitute for the usual breakfast fare. You'll find a number of wonderful pasta and rice dishes scattered throughout this book. Try them for breakfast.

Some good news—eggs, minus the bacon, are allowed! Fried eggs, scrambled eggs, poached eggs, hard-boiled, over easy, as omelets—the list goes on. We know the cholesterol in eggs is a nutritional bugaboo in some quarters these days. Our attitude is that unless you know you have a cholesterol problem, be good to yourself by not worrying unduly about eggs. Since you're allowed to have them, have them without guilt. Enjoy!

Try one or more of the following, sautéed in oil, with scrambled eggs: chopped onions, chopped tomatoes, chopped bell peppers; herbs such as parsley, chives, chervil, or tarragon. A garnish of caviar is fun. A side of salsa tastes and looks great with eggs. Eggs can be served on hot corn tortillas spread with margarine or butter. Other side dishes include broiled tomatoes and vegetables.

Here are some recipes we enjoy at breakfast:

🍂

RICE CEREAL WITH CINNAMON

Chris said, "Mary, this ain't a recipe—it's cereal with cinnamon."
Mary said, "I made it up, I cooked it—it's a recipe." So here it is:
Rice Cereal With Cinnamon.
 This is simplicity itself, and quite delicious. Find a packaged rice
cereal with no bad ingredients. Cereal should be cooked with water.

Packaged rice cereal   Margarine or butter
Cinnamon

Prepare cereal according to package directions. Add cinnamon and butter to taste.

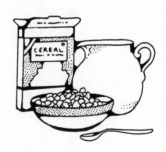

ᴈ

HOMINY GRITS

*Hominy is kernels of hulled dried corn with the germ removed. Grind them, and you have hominy grits. The following recipe is the basic preparation for this popular southern breakfast dish. If you buy your grits packaged, just follow the directions on the box. (**Note:** Packaged grits are much faster and easier to make.)*

We've never been a great fan of grits, or "gareeyuts" as they say in the South. But for a filling, fast breakfast, grits do the trick. When we eat them, we splurge on the margarine or butter, and add any flavor element that's handy: pine nuts, cinnamon, even onion. Grits take on the personality of whatever's available, so think of them as a blank culinary canvas and be creative.

1 cup grits	1 teaspoon salt
Water	Margarine or butter

Soak grits in water to cover for hour. Drain. Add 3 cups boiling water and salt. Cook gently for up to an hour. Cooking time varies depending on whether grits are ground fine, medium, or coarse. When grits are tender, they are done. Beat margarine or butter into hot grits if desired, and serve.

Serves 2

❧

MEXICAN BEANS

Beans for breakfast? Sure. They make a good accompaniment to Huevos Rancheros (page 44), or even plain old fried eggs, taking the place of toast. One of the up sides of this diet is that you get some relief from the boredom of having the same things for breakfast, day in, day out—toast, cereal, coffee...

2 tablespoons olive oil	1 29-ounce can pinto
2 garlic cloves, diced	beans

Heat the olive oil in a skillet. Add the garlic and cook gently for about 2 to 3 minutes — don't let it burn. Gradually stir in the liquid from the beans until the mixture thickens. Finally, add the beans. Mash half the beans and cook until everything is blended.

4 servings

??

BREAKFAST BURRITOS

Throw whatever's on hand into this one—chopped cilantro, pimiento, scallion....This is a good, hearty, healthy breakfast, but could use some flavor excitement. In the herb-and-spice section of your market, there's something called "Mexican Seasoning" which you can add while sautéeing. It will bring some additional character to the dish. Also try fresh salsas.

1 8-ounce can refried beans	1 small onion, chopped
1/2 cup cooked brown rice	1 teaspoon margarine or butter
1/2 cup ground turkey	4 to 6 corn tortillas
1 red pepper, diced	

Combine first five ingredients and sauté 5 minutes.

Spread margarine or butter on tortillas and zap in microwave. Or wrap in foil and heat 5 minutes at 350 degrees F. in oven or toaster oven. Wrap tortillas around bean mix and serve hot.

4 servings

ᴋ

BURRITOS WITH SCRAMBLED EGGS

One of the good things about moving to Southern California (Mary's from Wisconsin, Chris's from New York) was all the Mexican food we found here. It always seems not only to taste good but to be extremely wholesome and healthy as well. If chicken soup is "Jewish penicillin," maybe these breakfast burritos are "Hispanic Erythromycin."

1 small onion, minced
1 garlic clove, minced
2 tablespoons margarine or
    butter
2 small zucchini, diced
1/2 green pepper, diced

1 medium tomato, diced
7 eggs, beaten
Warm corn tortillas
Salsa (if desired)
Cilantro leaves

Sauté onion and garlic in butter until onion is soft, about 5 minutes. Add the zucchini, pepper, and tomato, and cook until the zucchini is tender. Stir until liquid evaporates. Pour in the eggs and scramble until the eggs are set.

Spoon egg mixture into warmed tortillas. Top with salsa. Garnish with cilantro leaves.

6 servings

HUEVOS RANCHEROS

This recipe is simple as can be, and absolutely delicious. It's one of our favorite breakfasts—very festive.

1 garlic clove, minced	1 pimiento, chopped
1 onion, chopped	3 tomatoes, chopped
3 tablespoons margarine or butter	8 eggs
	8 corn tortillas

Cook garlic and onion in 2 tablespoons of the margarine or butter until lightly browned. Add pimiento and tomatoes. Simmer until thickened.

In a separate pan, cook eggs sunny side up in remaining margarine or butter. Place each egg on a warmed tortilla and pour sauce over. Serve.

4 servings

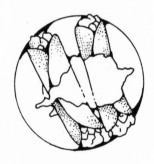

❧

EGGS BENEDICT

The challenge here is poaching the eggs so that they hold together. The usual way this is done is by adding a bit of vinegar to the poaching water. If you're not allergic to vinegar, we recommend this approach. If you don't want to add vinegar, try breaking each raw egg into a shallow cup, like a Japanese teacup, then upending it into the simmering water. Actually leave the cup in the water for 30 seconds or so, then remove. This can help hold the egg together, too. But vinegar is easier. If rice cakes are a little bland, try corn tortillas, or if you're one of those lucky few who are not allergic to wheat, splurge on some muffins.

Hollandaise Sauce (see   4 rice cakes
     page 160)   Margarine or butter
8 eggs

In a large skillet, simmer an inch of water. Add the eggs one at a time and poach 3 to 5 minutes.

Meanwhile, spread margarine or butter on rice cakes and set aside. Put two rice cakes on each plate.

Remove the eggs with slotted spoon and place two on each rice cake. Top with Hollandaise.

4 servings

❧

EGGS FLORENTINE

This recipe better be for one of your less tired mornings or very special days, like New Year's or Labor Day—it takes a while. The good news is it's lusciously delicious and will leave you feeling so undeprived you won't crave forbidden ingredients for a week.

1 cup rice	4 cooked artichoke bottoms (get the kind that's marinated in water)
1 small white onion, minced	
1 tablespoon margarine or butter	4 to 8 eggs
1 bunch spinach, well washed, trimmed, and chopped	Hollandaise Sauce (see page 160)
Pinch of nutmeg	Dash of paprika

Cook rice.

Sauté onion in margarine or butter. Add spinach and cook until soft, no more than 3 minutes. Add nutmeg, stir. Set aside and keep warm.

Poach eggs.

Put artichoke bottoms on hot plate, and spread with spinach mixture. Top each with one or two poached eggs. Add Hollandaise Sauce and a dash of paprika. Serve with heated rice.

4 servings

🐦

PIPERADE

This recipe goes back to the days when Chris and his carefree, twenty-something friends shared a summer house on Fire Island. They concocted this as a good breakfast after a night of carousing. They called it "piperade" because it contained tomato and thyme, like the French dish, and because Chris's friend Marylyn liked the word, either in its French pronunciation (peeper-odd) or in American (piper-ade, like a drink).

2 tablespoons oil	1/2 teaspoon thyme
2 medium onions, sliced	7 tablespoons margarine
4 garlic cloves, minced	or butter
1/2 bay leaf	12 eggs, lightly beaten
2 large tomatoes, peeled	Corn tortillas
and chopped	

Heat oil. Add onion, garlic, bay leaf, tomatoes, and thyme. Cook 15 minutes over low heat, stirring occasionally.

Meanwhile, melt margarine or butter in medium skillet and cook tortillas over low heat 2 minutes.

Add eggs to the onion mixture in the large skillet and cook, stirring over medium heat, until eggs thicken.

Put tortillas on warmed plates and cover with eggs.

6 servings

&&

GARLIC CORNMEAL CAKES

Eat these hot with plain or herb margarine or butter. Go ahead, slather it on—you've got enough dietary restrictions to worry about. Your kids, by the way, will enjoy these with pancake syrup.

1/4 cup margarine or butter	3 cups water
1 small onion, minced	1 1/4 cups cornmeal
1 garlic clove, diced	1 tablespoon olive oil

Preheat oven to 325 degrees F. Meanwhile, heat margarine or butter in a large saucepan, add onion, and sauté until soft. Add garlic and sauté for a minute. Add 3 cups of water and bring to a boil. Add the cornmeal, stirring constantly.

Cover and transfer the pan to the oven. Cook 25 to 30 minutes and serve. Or if you like, brush each square with a bit of the olive oil, then grill or broil, turning once, until cornmeal cakes are browned slightly, about 5 minutes.

6 servings

🦚

SPINACH TOMATO FRITTATA

Dirt is not on your diet, so wash the spinach well, plunging it into a bowl of cold water and draining, repeating this process until no more dirt comes away. Spinach, parsley, and leeks are the Pigpens of the vegetable world, always covered with dirt, so be sure to give them a good bath before you eat them.

3 tablespoons margarine or butter

1 pound spinach, all stems trimmed and rinsed

2 eggs, lightly beaten

1 tomato, seeded and diced

1 tablespoon minced onion

1 teaspoon minced garlic

1/4 teaspoon nutmeg

Preheat oven to 375 degrees F.

Melt margarine or butter in skillet. Stir in the spinach and cook for 4 minutes, until wilted. When cool enough to handle, chop and place in a bowl.

Grease a 9-inch pie pan. Stir eggs, tomatoes, onion, garlic, and nutmeg into the spinach. Spoon into the pie pan. Bake until batter sets, about 15 minutes.

Grease a baking sheet with margarine or butter. Invert the frittata onto a baking sheet, and remove the pie pan. Bake the frittata another 7 to 10 minutes, until completely done. Cut into wedges and serve.

4 servings

❧

CORN CASSEROLE

¹/₂ cup olive oil	2 cups frozen corn ker-
¹/₂ cup onion, chopped	nels, thawed
1¹/₂ cups fine chopped	2 egg yolks
green peppers	2 hard-boiled eggs,
1 large tomato, skinned	chopped
and chopped	¹/₄ teaspoon thyme

Preheat oven to 350 degrees F. In a skillet, heat ¹/₄ cup of the oil and sauté ¹/₄ cup of the onion and 1 cup of the green pepper until onion is tender. Add the tomato, and cook the mixture for 10 minutes. Then add the corn and egg yolks and cook, stirring, for an additional 3 minutes.

Heat the remaining oil in another skillet and sauté the remaining onion and green pepper until the onion is tender. Add the hard-boiled eggs and thyme and mix well.

Spread half the corn mixture in the bottom of a greased 1¹/₂-quart baking dish. Top with the hard-boiled egg mixture and then the remaining corn mixture. Bake about 15 minutes or until the corn is tender and the casserole is heated through.

4 servings

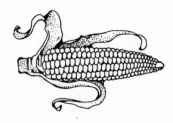

❧

MEXICAN STIR-FRY

This is a great breakfast dish because it's colorful enough to wake you up just looking at it. As a side benefit, it's delicious and healthily filling—it'll take you right through the morning.

1 tablespoon olive oil
2 garlic cloves, minced
1 medium onion, minced
2 small zucchini, diced
1 large sweet red pepper, diced
1 15½-ounce can garbanzo beans, rinsed and drained
1 15-ounce can black beans, rinsed and drained

½ cup water
¼ teaspoon oregano
2 tablespoons tomato purée
Warm corn tortillas
¼ cup cilantro leaves, chopped

Heat the olive oil in a wok or nonstick frying pan. Add the garlic, onions, zucchini, and red pepper. Stir-fry until the onions are tender, about 2 minutes. Add the garbanzo and black beans. Stir-fry an additional minute, and then add the water, oregano, and tomato purée. Stir-fry until hot, about 30 seconds. Serve with the warm tortillas; garnish with cilantro.

4 servings

❧

BREAKFAST STIR-FRY

This is a wonderfully filling meal. Include any intriguing leftovers you may have in the refrigerator. The mixture can be wrapped in warmed corn tortillas, if you wish.

This recipe probably takes longer to prepare than most breakfasts you're used to, but once it's cooked you have instant breakfast awaiting you for three additional days—six if you live alone.

1 chicken breast, skinned, boned, and cut into 1/2-inch chunks	2 tablespoons peanut oil
1 teaspoon minced fresh ginger	2 cups cooked rice, chilled
2 garlic cloves, minced	5 large scallions, sliced thin
1 tablespoon water	2 carrots, minced
2 teaspoons sesame oil	2 cups broccoli
	1/2 cup chicken broth

Cook rice and refrigerate the night before you plan to serve this dish. Mix chicken, ginger, garlic, water, and sesame oil together in a small bowl. Cover and refrigerate.

In the morning, heat 1 tablespoon of the peanut oil in a wok or nonstick pan over high heat. When very hot, add rice and half the scallions. Stir-fry over high heat for 2 minutes. Set aside in a large bowl.

Heat remaining oil. Add carrots and broccoli. Stir-fry until heated through, about 2 minutes. Add chicken broth and boil, stirring for 2 minutes, until vegetables are just tender. Add to the bowl.

Add chicken breast mixture to wok; stir-fry for a minute or so — the chicken cooks fast.

Pour contents of bowl back into the wok. Stir-fry until well mixed and heated through. Garnish with remaining scallions.

6 to 8 breakfast servings

🐌

STUFFED TOMATOES

5 large tomatoes
1½ cups falafel mix
2 tablespoons fresh parsley,
    chopped

1 tablespoon olive oil

Preheat oven to 350 degrees F.

Cut the tops off the tomatoes and scoop out the insides. Turn the shells upside down on paper towels to drain. Cut the seeded insides into chunks and set aside.

In a medium bowl, prepare the falafel mix according to directions. Stir in the tomato chunks and parsley.

Put the tomato shells in a shallow baking pan and stuff with the falafel mixture. Drizzle with olive oil. Bake for 15 minutes.

5 servings

✒

STUFFED PEPPERS

3 red peppers, cut in half
    and cleaned
1 small green pepper, cut
    in half and cleaned
4 tablespoons oil
1/2 cup quick-cooking rice
1 cup chicken broth
1/2 pound ground turkey

1 garlic clove, minced
3/4 cup chopped onion
1 tablespoon fresh or
    dried sage leaves,
    minced
2 tablespoons pine nuts,
    toasted

Place the red and green peppers skin side up on a broiler pan and broil until skins are slightly browned in spots and flesh is tender. Set red peppers aside. Dice green pepper when cool.

Put 1 tablespoon oil in a hot skillet, add the rice, and sauté about 2 minutes. Add the chicken broth and bring to a boil. Reduce heat to a simmer, and cook, uncovered, about 12 minutes, until rice is cooked and liquid has been absorbed.

Meanwhile, sauté turkey in remaining oil, stirring constantly until meat loses its pink color. Add the diced pepper, garlic, and onion, and continue cooking until turkey is done and vegetables are tender. Stir in the sage, pine nuts, and cooked rice. Heat thoroughly. Spoon mixture into red pepper halves.

6 servings

❧

KASHA AND SWISS CHARD

For people who think they don't like vegetables, this sensual eating experience could change a lot of minds—it's that voluptuous and flavorsome. If this dish were an actress, it would be Greta Scacchi. If an actor, possibly Tom Berenger.

4 large red Swiss chard
 stalks, trimmed
4 tablespoons margarine or
 butter
1/2 medium onion, chopped

1 cup chicken broth
1/2 cup whole kasha
 (a.k.a. buckwheat
 groats)
1 egg, lightly beaten

Cut chard leaves from ribs. Halve ribs lengthwise and slice thinly crosswise. Shred leaves. Melt 2 tablespoons of the margarine or butter in a heavy medium-size saucepan. Add onion and chard ribs. Cook about 10 minutes over moderate heat, stirring occasionally, until onion is tender. Add shredded leaves. Cook another 5 minutes. Add broth and bring to a boil.

Meanwhile, combine kasha and half the beaten egg in a bowl. Heat a large heavy skillet. Add kasha mixture and stir until egg dries and kasha kernels separate, about 3 minutes. Reduce heat to low. Add broth and vegetable mixture. Simmer covered until kasha is tender and liquid is absorbed—about 20 minutes. Add remaining margarine or butter and toss well.

2 servings

❧

CHIVE POLENTA

Other ingredients may be added to this polenta—corn kernels, chopped onion, red bell pepper in small dice, etc. Your imagination is the limit.

3 cups chicken broth
1¼ cups cornmeal
¼ cup chives, minced
2 tablespoons parsley,
    minced

3 tablespoons margarine
    or butter

Bring the stock to a boil in a large frying pan. Gradually whisk in the cornmeal. Lower heat and cook, stirring constantly, until mixture starts to thicken.

Immediately whisk in the chives, parsley, and two table-spoons of the margarine or butter. When the cornmeal has thickened, dot with the remaining tablespoon of margarine or butter.

You can serve the polenta as is or, for a special treat, broil it for a few minutes until golden brown. Or allow it to harden, slice it and sauté the pieces in olive oil.

4 servings

🕭

CHIVE POLENTA WITH SUN-DRIED TOMATOES

If you can find a packaged precooked polenta without bad ingredients, it makes this recipe a bit easier—you only have to stir it for 5 minutes. Use instead of cornmeal. We like Fattorie & Pandea Instant Polenta, which is imported from Italy and sold at most health food stores.

Our friend Paula, who kitchen-tested this recipe for us, says she prefers the polenta plain, without the tomato paste. But Paula enjoys making provocative statements—you should hear her go on about Bruce Springsteen. Anyway, we leave your choice of how to serve this to your personal taste buds.

3 cups chicken broth
1¼ cup yellow cornmeal
¼ cup minced chives
2 tablespoons minced
  parsley

3 tablespoons margarine
  or butter
Sun-dried tomato paste

Preheat broiler.

In a large, heavy, ovenproof pan, bring broth to a boil. Gradually whisk in the cornmeal. Cook, stirring often, until mixture pulls away from the sides of the pan—about 15 minutes.

Whisk in chives, parsley, and 1 tablespoon of the margarine or butter. Dot top of polenta with 1 tablespoon of margarine or butter.

Put the pan under the broiler and broil polenta until lightly browned—about 2 to 4 minutes. Let stand 5 minutes. Cut in wedges, then cut wedges in half lengthwise, and spread with the remaining margarine or butter and the sun-dried tomato paste.

2 to 4 servings

&ia;

SAUTÉED BROOK TROUT

*Sure, fish for breakfast. Dipped in cornmeal and cooked up fast,
nothing could taste better. And if you don't live in front of a lake,
the trout you can get at your supermarket is perfectly fine.*

2 to 4 trout, cleaned
½ cup cornmeal

2 tablespoons margarine
or butter

Choose the smallest, freshest fish available. Dip in cornmeal
to coat. Sauté in margarine or butter until browned on both
sides. Serve immediately.

2 servings

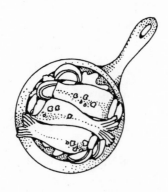

∽ 6 ∾

Lunch

Three possibilities here: away from home, home but tired, home and not so tired.

Away from home, pack some of Mary's Quickies, or eat at restaurants that have suitable foods—Middle Eastern, Mexican, or seafood. If you're at home, read on for some delicious and not-too-taxing recipes.

HOME BUT TIRED

"Sandwiches"

All right, these aren't exactly like the ones you get at the deli, but they taste delicious and don't take much time or energy to prepare.

Eat bread only if you're not allergic to anything in it: yeast, wheat, whatever. If you're not eating bread, corn tortillas are fine, wheat ones okay if you're allowed wheat. Rice cakes (made from whole-grain unprocessed rice) are fine, too, assuming they don't have cheese or some other no-no worked into them.

~

TUNA SALAD SANDWICH

1 small can tuna
½ cup Mayonnaise (see
    page 157) or health
    food alternative
¼ cup diced red onion

6 rice cakes
Margarine or butter
¼ cup chopped fresh
    parsley

Combine tuna, mayonnaise, and onion. Mix well. Spread rice cakes with margarine or butter. Top with tuna mixture. Garnish with parsley.

2 servings

Variations — add one or more of the following ingredients: chopped cilantro, chopped celery, curry powder, lemon juice, tomato slices, basil.

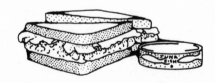

ᥰ

CHICKEN SALAD SANDWICH

When we were kids, all we ever had for lunch were three kinds of sandwiches: chicken salad, tuna salad, and peanut butter and jelly. How nice that two of them are still fine to eat, despite the diet. And we find that they still taste great, even unaccompanied by chocolate milk.

Meat from a cooked super-
  market chicken,
  chopped
1/2 cup chopped celery

3/4 cup Mayonnaise (see
  page 157) or health
  food alternative

Toss all ingredients in a bowl and spread on rice cakes or wrap in tortillas.

6 servings

Variations: Try with curry powder, lemon juice, and chopped basil leaves. Or tarragon, chopped cucumber, and chopped water chestnuts or walnuts.

❧

EGG SALAD WITH CUMIN

⅓ cup Mayonnaise (see
 page 157) or health
 food alternative
1 tablespoon lemon juice
¾ teaspoon ground cumin

6 hardboiled eggs,
 chopped
½ cup diced celery
¼ cup scallions, sliced
 thin

Mix all ingredients together in a bowl until well combined. Spread on rice cakes or wrap in heated tortillas.

About 2 cups

OTHER SANDWICH IDEAS

Grilled chicken breast with tarragon mayonnaise
Chopped shrimp with mayonnaise
Chopped lobster with mayonnaise
Hard-boiled egg, tuna, and mayonnaise
Sautéed eggplant with mayonnaise
Crabmeat with lemon juice and chives
Hard-boiled egg, onion, and mayonnaise
Hard-boiled egg, onion, raw spinach, and mayonnaise

HOME AND LESS TIRED

These soups, salads, burgers, and vegetarian dishes take a little longer, but all are good and on-target for your diet. Though we have arbitrarily put them into the lunch chapter, they of course taste just as good for dinner, or breakfast, or for midnight snacks. Lentil soup, for example, on a chilly morning, makes as good a breakfast as you could possibly imagine.

Soups

BEAN SOUP

4 cups chicken broth
½ cup sliced carrots
½ cup sliced onion
2 tablespoons lemon juice

3 cups white beans, cooked and drained, or canned white beans

Combine broth, carrots, onion, and lemon juice in a saucepan. Simmer, covered, until carrots are just tender. Stir in beans. Heat thoroughly.

4 servings

🐂

TIM'S BUTTERNUT SQUASH SOUP

This is a lush, velvety experience, a soup that's voluptuous. It was invented by our old pal, Tim, back in his Fire Island house days. Tim kept everyone fed no matter what madness was going on, and he always had a pot of something warm and nourishing on the stove.

2 tablespoons margarine or
    butter
2 tablespoons vegetable oil
2 cups chopped onion
1 3½-pound butternut
    squash, peeled, halved,
    seeded, and cut into
    ½-inch cubes

½ cup water
6 cups chicken broth

Heat margarine or butter and oil in a large skillet, add onion, and cook at low heat until soft, about 8 minutes. Add squash and water. Cook, covered, over moderately low heat for 30 minutes, until squash is tender. Add chicken broth and simmer, uncovered, for 15 minutes.

Process the soup in a blender or food processor in batches.

8 servings

Note: Soup may be made in advance and refrigerated.

❧

LENTIL SOUP

This humble lentil soup is great on chilly nights. All you need for accompaniment is a simple salad and some heated corn tortillas with margarine or butter. For those who are not allergic to wheat, substitute crusty bread for the tortillas. It's one of those dinners that tastes so healthy you think it'll cure you all by itself. It probably won't, but it sure won't hurt.

1 cup lentils
3 cups water
1 carrot, diced
2/3 cup onion, chopped
1 bay leaf
1/4 teaspoon ground thyme
2 tablespoons margarine or butter

1 pound tomatoes, chopped and seeded, or, on your low-energy days, 1 16-ounce can whole tomatoes, drained and chopped

Rinse lentils. Place in a pot with water, carrot, onion, bay leaf, and thyme. Bring to a boil over medium heat. Cover and simmer over low heat for 45 minutes. Add margarine or butter and tomatoes. Heat through. Serve.

4 servings

🐌

TOMATO-GARLIC SOUP

Peeling and seeding tomatoes doesn't have to be all that hard. Just heat a large pot of water to boiling, turn off the heat, and drop tomatoes in for a minute. (Italian plum tomatoes need to soak a minute longer—their skins are tighter.) Then pour tomatoes into a colander and spray with cold water to stop the cooking process. Now just cut tomatoes in half, and squeeze out the seeds and discard them. The seeds will pop out and the skin will pull off easily. The tomatoes will be ready for chopping.

4 medium garlic cloves,
  peeled and minced
2 tablespoons olive oil
2 pounds Italian plum
  tomatoes, peeled,
  seeded, and chopped

1¼ quarts chicken broth
6 basil leaves, chopped

In a large pot, sauté the garlic in the olive oil over low to moderate heat. Add the tomatoes and cook over low heat, uncovered, for about 10 minutes, stirring frequently.

Add the chicken broth and simmer for 20 minutes.

Stir in basil and serve. Or chill and serve, adding basil as garnish.

4 servings

❧

GAZPACHO

Yet another recipe from Fire Island. We were always having so much fun out there that we had to eat as healthily as possible to compensate for the havoc we were wreaking on ourselves. It must have worked, since we're all still around today.

1 carrot, peeled
2 scallions, each cut into
several pieces
1/4 red onion
2 cucumbers, peeled,
seeded, and cut in
chunks

Juice of 1/2 lime
3 pints cherry tomatoes
Chives, chopped

Purée carrot, scallions, red onion, cucumbers, and lime juice in a food processor or blender. Add the tomatoes and purée until gazpacho is the consistency of soup.

Chill. Serve in soup bowls garnished with the chopped chives.

6 servings

SPECIAL CHICKEN SOUP

A fine chicken soup. Nuff said.

6 cups chicken stock (or broth)

2 pounds boned chicken thighs, trimmed and cut into pieces

1/3 cup cooked nonwheat pasta

1 lemon or lime

2 eggs

1/2 cup cilantro, minced

Heat broth and add chicken pieces, bring to a simmer, and cook until the meat is done, about 5 minutes. Add the pasta, bring to a simmer, and remove from heat.

Squeeze 3 tablespoons of the lime or lemon juice into a bowl. Add the eggs and whisk together. Gradually add 2 cups of the broth to the egg mixture, whisking constantly. Slowly whisk the eggs back into the soup mixture.

Return to low heat until the soup starts to steam. Add cilantro and serve at once.

4 servings

❧

CARROT SOUP

Names of food items can be misleading. Here, this lush concoction, fit for kings and movie stars, is given the simple cognomen "Carrot Soup." Try it—we're not talking Campbell's. In fact, our friend Paula, who did try it, thought it was the best carrot soup she ever had—or imagined.

1 medium onion, sliced
  very thin
2 tablespoons margarine or
  butter
8 medium carrots, peeled
  and sliced ¼ inch thick

2 cups chicken broth
1 tablespoon peeled
  fresh gingerroot,
  minced fine
1 tablespoon fresh
  thyme leaves

In a large saucepan cook the onion in the margarine or butter until soft. Add the carrots and broth and simmer, covered, for 20 minutes.

Purée the carrots in batches in a food processor or blender. Transfer the purée to the saucepan, add the gingerroot and thyme, and simmer, stirring for 10 minutes.

Serve.

4 servings

❧

COLD AVOCADO SOUP

The key element here is lime juice. We've always been deeply impressed with limes—their color, their perfume, their fantastic flavor. As far as we're concerned, you can forget your fancy theological arguments—limes alone are sufficient proof of the existence of God. For this recipe, any lime will do, but get key limes if you can. They're sweeter.

4 avocados, mashed	4 cups chicken stock
Juice of 2 limes	Lime slices

Place mashed avocado and lime juice in food processor or blender, add some of the chicken stock and blend. Continue blending while adding the rest of the chicken stock until mixture is smooth and easy to pour. Add more lime juice to taste.

Chill soup. Garnish with lime slices when ready to serve.

8 servings

🐟

ONION SOUP

This is not the cheesy French onion soup, but a light, refreshing, and colorful American one. Makes a nice lunch or first course.

1 yellow bell pepper, cored, seeded, and cut into thin strips

3 tablespoons margarine or butter

2 leeks, trimmed, quartered lengthwise, and cut into 1/2-inch pieces

1 onion, diced

1 1/2 teaspoons fresh thyme

3 cups chicken stock

1 small tomato, peeled, seeded, and diced

Sauté pepper over low heat, maybe 20 minutes.

Meanwhile, heat the margarine or butter in a large pot over medium-low heat. Add the leeks and cook for 3 minutes. Add the onion and cook, stirring frequently, until soft, about 10 minutes. Stir in the thyme. Add the stock, bring to a boil, and simmer for 5 minutes.

Add the tomato and bell pepper to the soup and cook, over low heat, until just heated through.

4 servings

❧

AVGOLEMONO SOUP

This seems to be the national soup of Greece. It's seriously delicious. Isn't it great that we can give you great-tasting recipes like this so that you don't have to eat, for example, wheat germ and mashed tofu?

5 cups chicken broth	1/2 pound cooked
1 cup water	chicken, diced
1/4 cup instant rice	2 tablespoons fresh dill,
1/4 cup fresh lemon juice	chopped (optional)
3 eggs	

In a saucepan combine the chicken broth and water, and bring to a boil. Stir in the rice and cook according to directions on the box, or until soft.

In a bowl whisk together the lemon juice and eggs; whisk in 1 cup of the broth until fully mixed. Then whisk this mixture back into the remaining broth. Add the chicken and cook over medium-low heat, whisking, for 3 minutes. Do not allow to boil.

Serve, garnished with the dill.

6 servings

Salads

❧

SHRIMP AND CORN SALAD

This is great summer eating. Serve in a big lettuce leaf. Or in an avocado. You can even serve it in your bowling ball bag—it tastes great anywhere.

2 cups frozen corn kernels
1/2 pound small cooked
   shrimp
1 cup chopped celery
3 chopped scallions
1/4 teaspoon curry
   powder
Mayonnaise (see page
   157) or health food
   alternative

Cook corn according to package directions. Add the shrimp and remaining ingredients to the corn and stir well. Refrigerate for at least an hour before serving.

4 servings

ৰ্ক

CALIFORNIA SALAD

If you like the sort of food where sweet juicy things explode in your mouth, this recipe is for you. You can substitute red cherry tomatoes for the yellow ones. You can substitute lime juice for lemon juice. Just don't substitute regular onions for the red ones, or your friends will be calling you flame-breath for the rest of the night.

1 pound red tomatoes, cut into wedges
½ pound yellow cherry tomatoes, stems removed
½ cup fresh basil leaves

½ red onion, chopped
¼ cup extra-virgin olive oil
2 tablespoons lemon juice

In a large bowl combine red and yellow tomatoes, basil, onion, and oil, and toss well. Add lemon juice and toss again.

4 servings

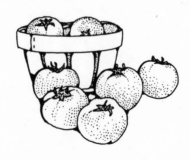

SQUID SALAD

1/3 cup lemon juice
1 tablespoon lemon peel, grated
1 1/4 cups light olive oil
1 1/4 pounds squid, cleaned and cut into rings
3 celery stalks, chopped
2 medium red bell peppers, quartered and cut into strips
2 tablespoons fresh basil, chopped

Put the lemon juice and lemon peel into a small bowl, and gradually whisk in 3/4 cup of the olive oil.

In a large skillet, heat 3 tablespoons of the remaining olive oil over high heat. Add the squid and tentacles and stir-fry until opaque, about 1 1/2 minutes. Transfer the squid to a colander. Add the remaining 2 tablespoons of olive oil to the skillet and reheat. Cook the celery, stirring until tender, about 2 minutes. Using a slotted spoon, add the celery to the squid. Next, fry the pepper strips until just soft, about a minute.

Return the squid and celery to the skillet. Add the basil and fry until just heated through. Put the mixture in a new bowl and add the dressing. Chill.

4 servings

❧

SEAFOOD SALAD

This is a fresh, delicious meal that's just right on a hot day. The prep work is a bit labor intensive—save time by buying the shrimp already cooked and not bothering to skin the tomatoes. We won't tell.

½ pound bay scallops
½ cup lime juice
3 dozen medium shrimp,
    cooked
2 medium tomatoes,
    unpeeled, chopped
1 onion, chopped fine

1 large avocado, peeled
    and cubed
3 tablespoons fine-
    chopped cilantro
6 large lettuce leaves
    (optional)

Put the scallops and lime juice in a large glass bowl. Marinate in the refrigerator for an hour. (The lime juice will "cook" the scallops.) Then add all other ingredients. Toss and serve in lettuce leaves if you wish.

6 servings

❧

EGGPLANT PASTA SALAD

This works two ways—warm as a pasta side dish, or cold as a salad, which was especially nice on the 100 + degree day we most recently cooked it.

5 tablespoons olive oil
4 Japanese eggplants, cut
   in ¼-inch slices
1 red pepper, cut in thin
   strips
1 yellow pepper, cut in thin
   strips
½ small red onion, cut in
   thin strips
1 medium garlic clove,
   crushed

½ cup basil leaves,
   chopped
1 8-ounce package
   quinoa pasta shells,
   cooked
3 tablespoons fresh
   lemon juice
¼ cup pine nuts, toasted
1 bunch arugula,
   chopped

In a large skillet, heat 2 tablespoons of the olive oil over medium heat. Cook the eggplant in batches until browned on both sides, adding more oil if necessary. Remove the cooked eggplant to a large bowl.

When all the eggplant is cooked, add the remaining olive oil to the skillet and sauté the peppers and onion until soft, about 5 minutes. Add the garlic and basil, and cook an additional 5 minutes.

Put the pepper mixture, cooked pasta, lemon juice, pine nuts, and arugula in the eggplant bowl and toss well.

6 servings

🎜

BARLEY-CORN SALAD

Man, have we ever learned about grains since we got on this diet. For us, barley was something that just never came up in our thoughts or recipes. But like so many of these exotic food items we've learned about, barley turns out to be soulful and delicious, and this is an extra-good salad. Give it a shot.

1 cup barley, rinsed well and drained	½ cup chopped fresh parsley leaves
1 cup chopped red bell pepper	2 tablespoons lemon juice
1½ cups corn kernels	⅓ cup olive oil

In a large saucepan of boiling water, slowly add barley and boil, stirring and skimming the froth, for about 30 minutes, or until barley is tender. Drain, rinse with cold water, and cool.

Transfer the barley to a large bowl and add pepper, corn, and parsley. In a small bowl mix lemon juice and oil, adding more lemon juice or oil depending on your taste. Toss salad with dressing.

6 servings

🐚

BLACK BEAN SALAD

We've learned to love black beans. In addition to this good salad, you can eat them just warmed up with maybe a little chopped onion in them, and some rice on the side. We serve them that way with mussels, which our eight-year-old unaccountably loves.

3 tablespoons lemon juice
1/3 cup olive oil
1-pound can black beans,
    drained, blanched in
    boiling water for 5
    seconds, and drained

1 cup chopped onion
2 tablespoons minced
    sun-dried tomatoes
2 cups romaine lettuce,
    rinsed, shredded,
    and chilled

Put the lemon juice in a bowl, and slowly add the oil, whisking until dressing is emulsified. Add beans, onion, celery, and tomatoes, and toss well.

Divide romaine lettuce onto four plates. Top with bean salad and serve.

4 servings

Fish

Fish is such a wonderful food. You can dress it up or down, and the possibilities are endless. For an easy lunch simply pan-fry or grill it; if you care for something a little more exciting—try these.

❧

CALAMARI WITH LIME AND GINGER

3 tablespoons Oriental
    sesame oil
3 tablespoons peanut oil
2 pounds squid, cleaned,
    cut into ¼-inch pieces
    (if possible, buy already
    cleaned and sliced; this
    is labor intensive, and
    some fish stores will do
    it for you)

2 scallions, chopped
2 tablespoons peeled
    fresh ginger, chopped
    fine
Juice of 1 lime
1 stick margarine or
    butter

Heat oils in a large skillet or wok. Add squid and sauté until opaque, about a minute. Remove squid to plate and keep warm. Add scallions, ginger, and lime juice to the pan, and boil down rapidly, scraping up any bits from the bottom of the pan. When the mixture is reduced by half, whisk in the margarine or butter. Serve squid with sauce poured over.

4 servings

❧

PAELLA

This dish will make you feel as if you've been living at the water's edge for nearly a month, in touch with the ebb and flow of the sea, and a simpler, better time.

However, it does cost more to make than the average dish in this book, and you may want to save it for a special feast. Our friend Leslie, who makes a world-famous gumbo, suggests adding some cayenne pepper. So if you're a hot mama like her, be our guest.

1 lobster
1/2 cup olive oil
2 garlic cloves, minced
1 frying chicken (2 to 3
    pounds), cut in small
    pieces
3 green peppers, sliced
4 medium onions, sliced
6 medium tomatoes, peeled
    and cut in wedges
3 cups uncooked rice

1/2 teaspoon saffron
Chicken stock
15 shrimp, cooked and
    shelled
15 mussels or clams,
    well scrubbed
2 cups green peas or
    sliced green beans
1 9-ounce package
    frozen artichoke
    hearts

Cook lobster until red. Remove meat. In a large skillet heat the olive oil and garlic. Sauté the lobster meat over medium heat for 2 or 3 minutes. Remove and reserve. Cook chicken until brown on all sides. Return lobster meat to skillet and add the green peppers, onions, and tomatoes. Cook for about 5 minutes, stirring constantly.

Add the rice and saffron and cook for another 5 minutes. Add chicken stock to cover, plus 1 inch. Cook, covered, over medium heat for 10 minutes, stirring occasionally. Add the shrimp, mussels, peas, and artichokes. Cover and cook for 10 minutes more or until the rice is tender, stirring frequently. If necessary, add more chicken stock, a little at a time. Cook until the paella is dry and all the liquid absorbed.

Serve hot.

8 to 10 servings

❧

SHRIMP KEBABS

Another of those simple grilled entrées we love so much. With this recipe, for instance, just paint some sliced zucchini, red bell pepper, and red onion with olive oil, and grill next to the shrimp. Start the veggies first, however, since they take longer to cook. Grill a little polenta next to them, and you've got a complete, delicious dinner.

20 ounces large shrimp, shelled and rinsed	1 small onion, grated
Juice of 3 lemons	1 garlic clove, minced
2 tablespoons olive oil	$1/8$ cup cilantro, chopped
	Cilantro sprigs

Place shrimp, lemon juice, and olive oil in a bowl. Marinate for 5 hours. Then add the onion, garlic, and chopped cilantro. Marinate for another hour.

Thread shrimp on skewers. Grill or broil until shrimp are done, 2 to 3 minutes. Entwine sprigs of cilantro on skewer and serve.

4 servings

❧

RATATOUILLE WITH SHRIMP

This is a more labor-intensive recipe than most. That's the bad news. The good is that it's unbelievably delicious and falls within the parameters of your diet.

A long, slow cooking process brings out unbelievable flavors in the vegetables. Remember, you'll need to start early. This is probably a Saturday meal rather than a Wednesday one.

1 large yellow onion, cut in
 1/2-inch thick slices
1/2 pound eggplant, cut in
 1/2-inch thick slices
1/2 pound zucchini, cut in
 1/2-inch thick slices
2 garlic cloves
2 green peppers, seeded
 and cut in strips
1 pound tomatoes, cut in
 1/2-inch slices

1 white onion, cut into
 1/2-inch slices
1/4 cup plus 1 tablespoon
 olive oil
1 pound shrimp, shelled
 and deveined
1/4 cup chopped fresh
 parsley

Layer yellow onion slices on the bottom of a large pot. Follow with a layer of eggplant and then one of zucchini. Mash the garlic and sprinkle over the zucchini. Continue layering with green peppers, tomatoes, and white onions. Repeat the layering until all vegetables are used. Drizzle 1/4 cup of oil on top and cover.

Bake at 250 degrees F. for 6 hours. Remove from the oven. Raise heat to 400 degrees F. Place the shrimp on top of the vegetables and drizzle with the remaining tablespoon of oil. Cover and bake for 10 minutes more. Garnish with parsley.

4 servings

❧

SWORDFISH SEVICHE

Good eatin' for hot weather—you don't have to heat up the kitchen.

8 ounces swordfish or
other fish steak, cut in
1/4-inch cubes
1/3 cup fresh lime juice
2 medium tomatoes,
peeled, seeded, and
diced

1/2 cup tomato juice
3 tablespoons olive oil
3 tablespoons fresh
oregano, chopped
coarse
1/2 bay leaf

Put swordfish in a large bowl, toss with lime juice, and
marinate in the refrigerator for an hour. Drain swordfish and
return to bowl. Add all remaining ingredients and toss well.
Cover and refrigerate for at least another hour.

4 servings

❧

PASTA WITH SHELLFISH AND HERBS

3 tablespoons lemon juice
3 tablespoons lime juice
1 pound scallops
2 lobsters (about 1¼ pounds each)
1 cup olive oil
6 scallions, chopped
1 tablespoon minced thyme
1 tablespoon minced basil
1 tablespoon minced oregano
¾ pound nonwheat angel-hair pasta, cooked

Combine juices in a large bowl, add the scallops, cover, and marinate in the refrigerator for an hour.

In a large pot, steam the lobsters in 1 cup of water over medium-high heat for 7 minutes. Drain and cool. Remove lobster meat from the shell and cut into scallop-size pieces.

Add the oil, lobster, scallions, scallops, juices, and herbs to the pasta, mix well, and refrigerate. Allow dish to marinate for an hour.

4 servings

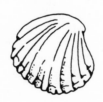

≈

CHINESE CALAMARI SALAD

3/4 cup sesame oil

3 tablespoons minced
   gingerroot

4 calamari fillets, cut into
   strips, or 10 whole
   cleaned squid, cut into
   rings

Juice of 1 lemon

1 1/2 heads of Belgian
   endive, chopped

1 bunch spinach, stems
   removed and
   chopped

1/4 teaspoon sesame
   seeds

"Vinaigrette" (see page
   157)

2 tablespoon vegetable
   oil

1 tomato, chopped

Combine sesame oil and ginger in a large bowl. Add the fish
and mix well. Cover and refrigerate overnight. Then add the
lemon juice.

Combine endive, spinach, and sesame seeds in a large
mixing bowl. Add 1/8 cup of "Vinaigrette" and mix well.
Remove fish from marinade and sauté quickly in hot
vegetable oil for about a minute. Place endive and spinach on
plates, and top with the calamari and tomatoes.

2 servings

❧

MONKFISH AND AVOCADO

Another tasty yet simple dish. Monkfish tastes a bit like lobster, so, if you're feeling daring and fancy-free, try lobster pieces instead of the fish.

1 12-ounce can tomato
   juice
2 tablespoons oil
1 tablespoon lime juice
1/4 teaspoon ground ginger
1 pound monkfish or
   swordfish, cut into
   1 1/2-inch pieces

1 avocado, peeled and
   cut into 1 1/2-inch
   pieces
1 tablespoon cornstarch
1 tablespoon chopped
   parsley

Mix together tomato juice, oil, lime juice, and ginger in a large bowl. Place fish in the marinade and refrigerate 1 hour, covered.

Remove fish from marinade, reserving marinade, and thread fish on skewers, alternating with avocado pieces.

Combine reserved marinade, cornstarch, and parsley in a 1-quart saucepan. Stir until blended. Cook over medium heat until slightly thickened, stirring constantly.

Broil fish until done, about 10 minutes, basting and turning frequently. Serve with sauce.

4 servings

Vegetarian Dishes

❧

VEGETABLE STIR-FRY

1/4 cup olive oil
3 garlic cloves, crushed
2 yellow bell peppers,
    cored and cut into
    1-inch pieces
2 red bell peppers, cored
    and cut into 1-inch
    pieces .
1 pound tomatoes, peeled,
    seeded, and chopped

1 10-ounce package
    frozen peas, thawed
    and drained
1 large onion, chopped
1/4 cup margarine or
    butter

Heat the oil in a wok or large skillet. Add garlic and stir until just brown. Add peppers and stir-fry for 2 minutes. Add tomatoes, peas, onions, and margarine or butter, and stir until heated through.

Transfer to a platter using a slotted spoon. Boil the remaining liquid until thick, about 5 minutes, then pour over vegetables. Serve on rice.

6 servings

🍃

EGGPLANT AND CHICKPEA CASSEROLE

Chris's first awareness of chickpeas came at the notorious New York nightspot of the sixties and seventies, Max's Kansas City. There was a dishful on every table, and you could watch the celebrities and drug addicts snacking on them. Rest assured, though, this recipe is very wholesome, another of those soulful vegetarian meals that you think will heal you all by themselves. Try it.

1/4 cup plus 2 tablespoons vegetable oil
1 1/2 teaspoons cumin seed
1/2 teaspoon fennel seeds
2 medium onions, sliced
12 large garlic cloves, sliced thick
2 teaspoons dried mustard
1 teaspoon curry powder

1 small eggplant, unpeeled, cut into 1/2-inch-thick-by-2-inch-long pieces
5 fresh plum tomatoes, quartered lengthwise
1 19-ounce can chickpeas, rinsed and drained
2 tablespoons fresh cilantro, chopped

In a large skillet, heat oil over high heat. Add cumin seed and cook until dark brown, about 15 seconds. Add fennel seeds and cook for 5 seconds more. Then add the onion and garlic and reduce heat to medium-high. Cook, stirring often, for 5 to 10 minutes, until the onion and garlic are tender.

Stir in the mustard, curry, and eggplant. Add more oil if necessary. Reduce heat to moderate and cook, stirring gently, until eggplant is limp, about 5 minutes. Add the tomatoes and cook, stirring constantly, until soft, about 5 minutes. Gently stir in the chickpeas, cover, and simmer over low heat until liquid is thickened, about 5 minutes.

Sprinkle cilantro on top and serve.

6 servings

🐌

EGGPLANT CURRY

You say you're too tired to deal with cooking a recipe tonight? Try this: Cut that eggplant you bought into ¹/₂-inch slices. Paint with a good olive oil. Grill or broil until golden brown. Eat. Roll eyes in pleasure. Watch TV.

1 large eggplant	1 garlic clove, sliced
1 onion, sliced thin	1 large tomato, chopped
1 tablespoon olive oil	3 tablespoons cilantro,
1 teaspoon cumin	chopped
¹/₂ teaspoon turmeric	

Preheat oven to 400 degrees F.

Pierce the eggplant with a fork, then bake for 1 hour at 400 degrees F. Remove from the oven, slice open, and let liquid drain for 30 minutes. Then cut eggplant flesh into 1-inch cubes.

Meanwhile, sauté the onion in olive oil over medium-high heat until golden brown. Add cumin, turmeric, and garlic. Sauté an additional minute, then add tomato and cook on high until most of the liquid is gone. Add eggplant and cilantro. Heat through.

4 servings

❧

EGGPLANT WITH MARINARA SAUCE

This is as delicious a recipe as you'll find in this whole book. Sweet, luscious, flavorful—really a knockout. Eggplant and olive oil are one of God's great flavor combinations. If you're in a hurry, or feeling tired, just grill or broil the slices painted with olive oil— forget the sauce. They're delicious just like that.

1 large eggplant, sliced thin
Olive oil
1 cup Marinara Sauce (see page 161)
2 large tomatoes, sliced thin

8 ounces soy cheese, sliced thin
Fresh or dried basil leaves
Fresh or dried oregano leaves

Preheat oven to 350 degrees F.

Prepare eggplant slices by painting them with a good olive oil and either broiling or grilling them. You may also sauté them in olive oil. Slices are done when they are browned.

Pour half of the Marinara Sauce in a shallow baking dish. Put eggplant slices in the dish and place a tomato slice and a cheese slice on top of each eggplant slice. Cover with remaining Marinara Sauce and season with basil and oregano leaves. Heat in the oven for 5 to 10 minutes—until heated through.

8 servings

🕿

THIRTY-MINUTE RATATOUILLE

We find that with most ratatouille recipes the more you cook them, the better they taste. It has something to do with the melding of all the subtle vegetable flavors. But if you don't have the time or inclination for lengthy cooking, try this recipe—the short version. It's really good. Still, if you're hankering for that extra flavor and texture, all you have to do is let this simmer a while longer. This also is one of those dishes that taste better the next day.

2 red bell peppers, cored
    and cut into strips
2 green bell peppers, cored
    and cut into strips
1/4 cup olive oil
2 zucchini, sliced

1 small eggplant, halved
    lengthwise and sliced
1 onion, sliced
Chopped fresh cilantro
    to taste

Sauté the peppers in a wok or large skillet in 1 tablespoon of the olive oil until tender, about 3 or 4 minutes, then remove. Add another tablespoon of the olive oil and stir-fry zucchini until browned, about 3 or 4 minutes, then remove. Add another tablespoon of the olive oil and stir-fry eggplant slices until browned, about 3 or 4 minutes; then remove.

Heat the remaining tablespoon of olive oil and stir-fry onion slices 3 minutes until browned. Add all the reserved vegetables and the cilantro, and heat through.

6 servings

ع❧

VEGETABLE SKILLET

For you folks who think vegetarian food is something that leaves you hungry again a half hour later, try this—it sticks to your ribs. What you are essentially doing with the eggs is poaching them in the pan juices. It may take a little longer to do this than you might expect, so be patient. Then serve…and break the yolks so they run all over the food. Seriously delicious.

2 teaspoons olive oil
1 onion, minced
1 garlic clove, minced
1 eggplant, peeled and chopped into cubes
1 leek, carefully washed and cut into thin slices

2 tomatoes, peeled and diced
4 eggs
Chopped parsley

Heat the olive oil in a large skillet. Add the onion and garlic. Sauté until onion is tender. Add the eggplant, leek, and tomatoes. Stir well. Reduce heat, cover, and simmer for 20 minutes.

Uncover. Using bottom of large spoon, make four "nests" in the cooking vegetables. Break eggs into nests. Simmer until eggs are poached to desired doneness, sprinkle with parsley, and serve.

4 servings

❧

CABBAGE AND TOMATO CURRY

This is one of our favorite recipes in the book. The cabbage has a wonderful crunchy texture, and the spices are delicious. We could eat this every night.

When you add the cabbage, you may think you've chopped up too much—it seems to make a small mountain in the pan. Don't worry, it cooks down fast.

1 tablespoon oil	3/4 white cabbage, chopped
1 1/2 teaspoons black mustard seeds (use plain mustard seeds if you can't find these)	1 onion, chopped
	3 tomatoes, coarsely chopped
1/4 teaspoon fennel seeds	1 tablespoon minced cilantro
1 tablespoon curry powder	

Heat the oil in a large skillet over high heat. Add the mustard seeds and sauté until hot. Then add the fennel seeds, browning slightly. (These operations don't take long.) Add the curry powder, cabbage, and onion. Sauté for 5 minutes. Finally add the tomatoes and cilantro, stirring occasionally, until sauce is thickened. Serve as a side dish, or over rice as a vegetarian dinner.

4 servings

∽ 7 ∾

Dinner

In most households, including ours, dinner is the one meal of the day when there's a little more time to make things nice, and a little more time to sit down and enjoy it. So don't just eat more rice cakes with nut butter—dine.

The idea is to put a protein, a vegetable, and a grain on your plate, desirably all at the right temperature and degree of doneness. Simple, but complete and perfect.

Vegetables

The most simple, direct, delicious, and wonderful way to eat vegetables is steamed and tossed with margarine or butter and herbs.

How long this takes depends on the vegetable. Snap peas cook in 3 minutes, artichokes can take as long as 45. Most take 10 to 15 minutes. In general, your vegetable is at the right degree of doneness when the tines of a fork are *just* beginning to slip in easily.

Herbs wonderfully enhance vegetables. Chop them and allow them to sit awhile in hot margarine or butter or olive oil. Accompanying them with herbs makes eating vegetables a truly sensual experience. Here are some good combinations:

Vegetable	*Accompaniment*
Artichokes	margarine or butter, garlic margarine or butter, Hollandaise Sauce (see page 160)

95

Asparagus margarine or butter, lemon juice,
Hollandaise Sauce

Beets margarine or butter, dill, chives,
thyme, lemon juice, orange
peel

Broccoli margarine or butter, dill,
rosemary, lemon juice, chopped
sun-dried tomatoes

Brussels sprouts margarine or butter, basil, chives,
dillweed, minced parsley,
rosemary, thyme, chopped
pecans

Carrots margarine or butter, basil, chives,
dillweed, ginger, mint, nutmeg,
minced parsley, lemon juice

Cauliflower margarine or butter, chives,
dillweed, nutmeg, minced
parsley, lemon juice,
Hollandaise Sauce

Corn margarine or butter, margarine or
butter with curry powder, lime
squeezed over

Cucumbers margarine or butter, chervil,
chives, dillweed, minced
parsley

Eggplant garlic margarine or butter, basil,
oregano, marjoram, minced
parsley

Green beans	margarine or butter, dillweed, thyme, chives
Okra	margarine or butter, lemon juice, chopped chives, minced parsley
Peas	margarine or butter, nutmeg, tarragon, chives, thyme
Spinach	margarine or butter, nutmeg, grated lemon peel
Squash (summer)	margarine or butter, basil, oregano, dillweed
Squash (winter)	margarine or butter, nutmeg, cinnamon
Sweet potatoes	margarine, lemon peel and juice, chopped pecans, cinnamon, nutmeg
Swiss chard	hot margarine or butter, basil, nutmeg, oregano
Turnips	hot margarine or butter, basil, dill, caraway seeds

Here are some other wonderful vegetable dishes that are on target for your diet:

❧

CINNAMON PARSNIPS

*So simple, so good. And you have the fun of watching your guests'
stunned expressions when they ask you what vegetable that is, and
you tell them. Wow, they'll think, someone who knows about
parsnips.*

1/2 pound parsnips, peeled,   1/2 teaspoon cinnamon
    trimmed, and shredded
2 tablespoons margarine or
    butter, softened

Steam the parsnips in a vegetable steamer, covered, for 3
minutes or until just tender.

In a heated bowl toss parsnips with margarine or butter
and cinnamon.

2 servings

✿

SPAGHETTI SQUASH

Mmm—nicely goopy. Puts that little sensual hit in your evening. Since spag-squash, as we call it, is relatively bland, you can think of it as a canvas to make individual and beautiful art upon. Try a dash of nutmeg, or chopped scallions, or toasted pine nuts, or chopped sun-dried tomatoes...

1 spaghetti squash	1 garlic clove, pressed
Butter or margarine to coat squash, plus 2 tablespoons	1 teaspoon chopped fresh oregano (dried can be used)

Prepare the spaghetti squash according to the directions on the accompanying tag. If it has no directions, cut in half lengthwise, clean out the innards, and spread the squash liberally with margarine. Put plastic wrap over both halves, put in microwave, and cook at 5-minute intervals, turning each time, until squash is relatively soft, about 10 to 12 minutes.

While the squash is cooking, melt the 2 tablespoons of margarine or butter in a small skillet. Add garlic and oregano and cook over low heat for 10 minutes.

When squash is finished, open and make "spaghetti." Toss with margarine or butter mixture and serve.

4 servings

🐌

ZUCCHINI AND PEPPER MIX

1 tablespoon margarine or
   butter
1 red bell pepper, cut into
   ½-inch pieces

½ pound zucchini, sliced

In a large skillet, add margarine or butter and cook the pepper, covered, over medium-low heat for 5 minutes, stirring occasionally. Add zucchini and cook, stirring occasionally, for 6 minutes or until zucchini is tender.

2 servings

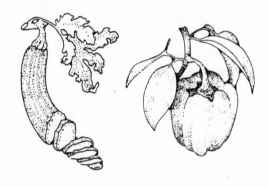

🖤

FENNEL AND LEEKS

1 large fennel bulb,
    chopped into 1/4-inch
    pieces
12 garlic cloves, peeled
1 tablespoon extra-virgin
    olive oil

4 medium leeks (about 1
    pound), chopped
    into 1/4-inch pieces

Preheat oven to 450 degrees F. Place a sheet of heavy-duty aluminum foil about 2 feet by 1 foot on a work surface. Arrange fennel and half the garlic cloves on one half of foil. Drizzle with 1/2 tablespoon of the olive oil. Fold empty half of the foil over fennel and crimp the edges to form a tight seal. Place the package on a baking sheet.

Do the same with the leeks, placing them and the 6 remaining garlic cloves on a large sheet of aluminum foil. Drizzle with remaining olive oil. Fold the foil over, seal, and place package on the same baking sheet with fennel.

Bake vegetables for 10 minutes. Then flip the packages over and bake for 15 more minutes. Remove from the oven and let stand without opening for 5 minutes. Remove vegetables from foil and mix together in a medium bowl. Serve.

This can be served warm or put in the refrigerator and served at a later time, chilled.

4 servings

ஜ

BRAISED FENNEL

We discovered fennel one day when we were playing baseball in a vacant lot with our hip friends Eva and Rex. Someone whacked the ball into an anonymous patch of greenery—and this fabulous licorice scent suddenly ravished us. It turned out fennel just grows wild, and we were able to dig up a few bulbs and braise them. It was love at first smell—and taste.

The more margarine or butter you whisk in at the end, the more sumptuous things become. This is an unabashedly sensual dish. You could be excommunicated for eating braised fennel.

6 medium fennel bulbs with fronds	1/4 cup margarine or butter or olive oil
1 smallish onion, sliced	1 cup chicken broth
1 garlic clove, minced	1 sprig thyme
1 small carrot, grated	Up to 3 tablespoons of margarine or butter
Few celery leaves, chopped	

Discard fennel fronds, and quarter the bulbs. Sauté onion, garlic, carrot, and celery leaves in margarine or butter.

Sauté fennel quarters on all sides. Add broth and thyme sprig. Bring to a boil, reduce heat, cover, and simmer until fennel is tender, about 25 minutes. Test with fork for doneness.

Remove fennel to warmed serving dish; tent with foil. Boil down pan liquids by two-thirds or more, until somewhat thick. Discard thyme sprig. Whisk in margarine or butter to taste.

6 servings

❧

BEET AND PARSNIP FRY

Does this recipe strike anyone as a little, well, off the beaten path? Possibly it's been some time since you hazarded a parsnip. Well, we guarantee you a major taste treat here. Really, there were four grown people at our table one night fighting for the last helping. And these were people who had earlier exclaimed "Beet and Parsnip Fry? Eyew!" You could say this recipe falls into the mind-blower category.

1 medium beet, unpeeled
1 medium parsnip, peeled
  and grated
1/4 teaspoon dried thyme,
  crumbled

3 tablespoons margarine
  or butter
1 tablespoon minced
  shallot
Fresh thyme sprigs

Preheat oven to 350 degrees F. Place the beet in a small baking pan and bake until tender, about an hour. Grate and toss with parsnip and thyme.

Melt 1 tablespoon of the margarine or butter in a heavy skillet over medium heat. Add shallot and stir for 30 seconds. Then add the beet-and-parsnip mixture and cook for 3 minutes.

Add the remaining 2 tablespoons of the margarine or butter and cook over low heat, stirring occasionally, for 10 minutes. Sprinkle with thyme sprigs and serve.

2 servings

❧

BRAISED ROOT VEGETABLES

This is one of our favorite vegetable recipes. It's a standby on Thanksgiving, and all through the winter months. It's so delicious our guests freak out. "This is great," they cry out, and demand the recipe. Whether they get it or not depends on if they're willing to help clean up. But you get it for free!

1/4 cup margarine or butter
4 garlic cloves, peeled
1 onion, sliced
1/2 pound carrots, peeled and cut into diagonal pieces
1 pound sweet potatoes, peeled and sliced thick

1/2 pound parsnips, peeled and cut into diagonal pieces
2 tablespoons chopped parsley

Melt half the margarine or butter in a large skillet. Add garlic and onions, and cook until tender. Then add carrots, potatoes, parsnips, and water to cover. Bring to a boil. Simmer covered until vegetables are just tender but not mushy, about 20 minutes.

Uncover and bring to a rapid boil. When liquid has evaporated, add remaining margarine or butter in pieces, stirring so vegetables are fully coated, and sprinkle with parsley.

6 servings

🐌

BRUSSELS SPROUTS AND CARROTS

1 pound Brussels sprouts,
  trimmed and cut in half
1 pound carrots, peeled
  and cut in half
  lengthwise and then
  crosswise
⅓ cup margarine or butter

1 teaspoon caraway
  seeds
1 garlic clove, minced
Grated peel of 1 lemon
2 tablespoons lemon
  juice

In a large skillet, cook Brussels sprouts and carrots in an inch of boiling water, until tender, about 10 to 15 minutes. Drain well.

In the same pan, melt the margarine or butter and add the caraway seeds, garlic, lemon peel, and lemon juice. Add the cooked vegetables and heat.

6 servings

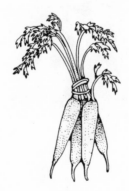

&

SAUTÉED EGGPLANT

Elegant, straightforward, fine. How to put nice vegetables on your plate without straining.

2 tablespoons olive oil   1 garlic clove, minced
1 Japanese eggplant, sliced   1 tomato, chopped
   thin

Add the olive oil to a large skillet and sauté eggplant until browned on both sides. Drain on paper towels.

In the same pan, sauté garlic, then add the tomatoes and cook until soft. Add the eggplant and reheat.

2 servings

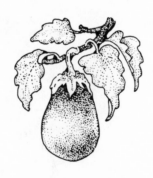

🐦

BRAISED KALE

We love Greens. No, not that German political group—though they seem very nice, too—but all these things like collards, kale, beet greens, chard, and so forth. Very, very healthy. And with a kind of soulful quality that's very appealing. Try these.

1 tablespoon margarine or butter	1 pound kale, stems discarded, leaves chopped
1 small onion, chopped fine	1 tablespoon lemon juice

In a large skillet, melt the margarine or butter, and sauté the onion until tender, about 5 minutes.

Meanwhile, rinse the kale in cold water, add it to the skillet, and simmer covered 15 to 20 minutes, stirring occasionally.

Sprinkle with lemon juice.

4 servings

❧

BRUSSELS SPROUTS WITH PECANS

³/₄ cup pecans, minced   2 pounds Brussels
4 tablespoons margarine or   sprouts
  butter

Cook pecans over low heat in margarine or butter until lightly
browned, about 15 minutes.

Wash Brussels sprouts. Trim off outside leaves. Steam
until tender.

Put the pecan margarine or butter and Brussels sprouts in
a large frying pan and heat through, stirring occasionally.

4 to 6 servings

❧

ZUCCHINI GREEK STYLE

3 tablespoons olive oil   2 tomatoes, skinned and
1 garlic clove, minced   chopped
1 small onion   ¹/₂ teaspoon oregano
1 pound zucchini, in   1 tablespoon chopped
  ¹/₄-inch slices   parsley

Heat the oil in a large skillet. Sauté garlic and onion until
tender.

Add zucchini and simmer, covered, until almost tender,
about 5 minutes. Stir in tomatoes, oregano, and parsley.
Simmer 2 more minutes.

4 servings

Grains and Beans

Once again, we'll assume you know the rudiments of cooking rice and beans or have cookbooks that can teach you.

Rice made with chicken broth is more sumptuous than with water.

Check out the good boxed rice and grain dishes available at health food stores. Many of them are delicious and dietetically correct. See examples in chapter 3—Shopping.

Also, don't forget lentils. They are healthy, cheap, and easily prepared...in countless delicious ways.

🍃

WILD RICE

Crunchy. That's what a lot of rice dishes should be and aren't. This never-fail-to-get-a-compliment wild rice recipe is a super-delicious crowd-pleaser.

1/4 pound wild rice	1/2 piece celery, minced
2 1/2 cups water	2 tablespoons margarine
1/4 cup pine nuts	or butter
Half a medium onion, minced	1/2 cup chicken stock

Cook rice in water over low heat for 50 minutes or until tender, and then drain.

In a saucepan sauté pine nuts, onion, and celery in margarine or butter over medium heat for 10 minutes. Add rice and chicken stock and cook, stirring, until chicken stock is absorbed, about 5 to 10 minutes.

2 to 4 servings

≈

SPICY WILD RICE

And for those of you who'd like this to actually be spicy, as its name suggests, better add some salt and pepper.

2 tablespoons margarine or butter	1 leek, carefully washed and diced
1 carrot, diced	2 cups wild rice
1 celery stalk, diced	4 cups chicken stock

Heat margarine or butter over medium-low heat. Add carrot, celery, and leek. Cook, stirring occasionally, for about a minute. Stir in rice and add the chicken stock; cover, and cook slowly until rice is done, about 1 hour and 15 minutes. Add extra chicken stock as needed.

8 servings

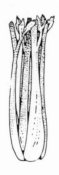

❧

RED BEANS AND RICE JOHNNY OTIS

This is labor-intensive. It is, however, nutritionally complete, so if you make it, you won't have to cook anything else that night. And it's much easier with canned kidney beans; you won't need to soak them overnight. Use two 16-ounce cans of kidney beans—that's roughly equivalent to a pound of dried beans.

We got into red beans and rice thanks to rhythm-and-blues progenitor Johnny Otis, who throws an annual "Red Beans and Rice Cookoff" here in California, featuring great soul and blues artists. So we're naming our recipe after him. Thanks, Johnny.

Beans:

1 pound dried red kidney beans	4 garlic cloves, minced
2 cups chopped onion	4 cups chicken stock
¼ cup olive oil	2 bay leaves

Rice:

2 tablespoons olive oil	2 cups long-grain rice,
½ cup chopped onion	freshly cooked

Beans: Place beans in a bowl, cover with water, and let soak for 24 hours. Drain and set aside.

In a large saucepan sauté onion in olive oil over low heat until golden brown, about 15 minutes. Add garlic and sauté another 3 minutes. Add beans and stock and bring to a boil. Reduce heat, cover, and simmer for 2 hours. Add bay leaves, cover, and continue simmering until beans are tender, about another hour. Transfer to a bowl and keep warm.

Rice: Heat oil in a large skillet over medium-low heat. Add the onion and sauté until tender, about 10 minutes. Add the rice and heat through.

Serve rice and beans side by side or place the rice in bowls and top with beans.

6 servings

❧

LENTIL PILAF

Don't rice and lentils and stuff taste healthy? *And, in fact, they are! But what's great is they're* deliciously *healthy.*

1 bunch scallions, chopped
2 garlic cloves, minced
1 cup lentils, rinsed
1/2 cup brown rice, rinsed
1/4 cup wild rice, rinsed
1/4 cup margarine or butter

2 tablespoons slivered
  almonds
1/2 teaspoon dried thyme
  leaves, crushed
2 1/2 cups chicken broth

In a large skillet, sauté the scallions, garlic, lentils, and both rices in margarine or butter until the onion is tender, about 4 minutes. Add the almonds, thyme, and chicken broth, and bring to a boil. Reduce heat and simmer, covered, for about 30 minutes or until the liquid is absorbed.

6 servings

ᥲ

MARY'S CASSOULET

Labor-intensive, but worth it. Save effort by using canned white beans—two 16-ouncers ought to do it. Great Northern's good.

This gets five yums on the yum scale. It's a real cassoulet, with hearty flavors that are a perfect match with cool autumn evenings and a fire in the fireplace.

1 pound dry white beans	5 chicken thighs
1 carrot, sliced	2 tablespoons oil
1/4 teaspoon dried thyme	1/2 cup onion, chopped
1 onion, studded with 6 cloves	2 garlic cloves, minced
1/4 pound veal	3 tablespoons margarine or butter

Soak beans overnight in water, making sure the water covers the beans. The next day add the carrots, thyme, and whole onion studded with cloves to the pot. Stir. Bring the mixture to a boil, reduce heat, and simmer, covered, for 1 1/2 hours. Add more water if needed.

Place the veal in a small pan, cover with boiling water, and cook for 10 minutes. Remove from the pan, dice, and add to the beans.

Put the oil in a large frying pan, add the chicken, and sauté until well browned. Remove the chicken and set aside. Add the onions and garlic to the pan and cook in remaining drippings until tender.

Add the onion-and-garlic mixture to the beans. Layer beans and chicken in a 3-quart casserole. Dot the top with butter or margarine. Cover and bake at 250 degrees F. for 3 hours, adding water as needed if cassoulet becomes too dry.

4 servings

Pasta

The bad news about pasta is that it's generally made from wheat and wheat is allowed only if you're not allergic to it. The good news is there are now pastas available made from a mixture of quinoa, a South American grain that's on your approved list, and corn flour, which for many people is not a problem. The brand we found is Ancient Harvest, which comes in several shapes. Look for quinoa, amaranth, and corn pasta, as well as Japanese buckwheat noodles, at your local health food store. Remember, vegetable noodles are mainly wheat and should be introduced only when you've started the Phase Two diet.

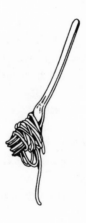

❧

PASTA WITH TOMATO BASIL SAUCE

Simple. Easy. Delicious. Recipes like this are what this book is about.

1 pound pasta	1 teaspoon parsley,
1/2 cup olive oil	chopped
6 garlic cloves, puréed	1/2 cup soy cheese,
6 large tomatoes, diced	crumbled
2 tablespoons basil,	3/4 cup toasted pine nuts,
chopped	optional

Cook the pasta in boiling water, according to package directions, until *al dente*. Drain. Add 1 tablespoon of the olive oil and stir.

Meanwhile, sauté half the garlic in a large skillet using 2 tablespoons of the olive oil. Cook over medium heat for about a minute. Add the tomatoes and basil. Bring to a boil, reduce heat, and simmer for 40 minutes or until the sauce begins to thicken.

In a separate pan, sauté the remaining garlic in the remaining olive oil. Cook for about a minute. Add the pasta and toss over high heat until heated through. Sprinkle with cheese and most of the parsley and mix well. Transfer to a hot serving platter. Top with tomato sauce. Garnish with pine nuts and remaining parsley.

6 servings

❧

PASTA AND TUNA

Simple, easy, good. They sell olive-oil-packed tuna in Italian delis. If you have the kind packed in water, add a bit of good-tasting olive oil that you keep in your cabinet for moments like this.

3 tablespoons olive oil
1 large onion, chopped
3 scallions, minced
2 6½-ounce cans tuna
    packed in oil
3 cups tomato sauce

¼ cup chopped green
    pepper
3 tablespoons chopped
    fresh parsley
1 pound nonwheat pasta

Heat the oil in a large pot, add the onion and scallions and sauté until golden. Stir in tuna, with its own oil, breaking into small pieces. (If tuna is packed in water, discard water and add another tablespoon of olive oil.)

Cook over medium heat for 2 minutes. Cool for a moment, then add the tomato sauce, pepper, and 1 tablespoon of the parsley. Simmer for 5 minutes, then remove from heat and let stand while cooking the pasta.

Cook the pasta in 6 quarts of boiling water until *al dente*. See package directions for cooking time, or test from time to time. Drain thoroughly in a colander. Put pasta on plates; top with sauce. Sprinkle with remaining parsley.

4 servings

✒

PASTA WITH RED AND GREEN PEPPERS

We also cook this with red and yellow peppers instead of the green ones, which makes for a sweeter, more succulent meal. It's even better if you roast the peppers first, but if you don't feel like it, the dish is just fine with the peppers sautéed.

1/2 pound nonwheat pasta
2 tablespoons margarine or butter
2 tablespoons olive oil
8 sun-dried tomatoes, packed in oil, chopped
1/4 cup fresh basil
1/4 cup chopped fresh parsley
4 garlic cloves, minced
2 sweet red peppers, cut in strips
2 green peppers, cut in strips

Following package directions, cook the pasta in boiling water unti *al dente.* Drain.

Meanwhile, in a saucepan heat margarine or butter and olive oil. Add the tomatoes, basil, parsley, garlic, and peppers. Sauté until heated through.

Add the pepper-and-tomato mixture to the pasta and mix well.

4 servings

❧

LENTILS AND PASTA

This dish defines "earthy." We mean that in the best possible sense.

1 cup dried lentils
4 cups water
2 tablespoons olive oil
1 cup onions, chopped fine
3 garlic cloves, minced

2 teaspoons ground
  cilantro
½ pound pasta
3 tablespoons margarine
  or butter

Boil the lentils and water in a medium saucepan. Reduce heat and simmer, uncovered, until lentils are tender, about an hour. Add more water as needed. Drain.

Meanwhile, heat the olive oil in a large skillet. Add the onions, garlic, and cilantro, and sauté until the onion is tender, about 10 minutes.

Following package directions, cook the pasta in boiling water until *al dente*. Drain.

Put the pasta, lentils, and margarine or butter in a large skillet. Cook over low heat, stirring occasionally, until margarine or butter is melted. Add the onion mixture, heat thoroughly, and serve.

6 servings

PASTA WITH CRAB SAUCE

4 ounces nonwheat
  spaghetti
1 tablespoon margarine or
  butter
1/2 cup scallions, chopped
1 garlic clove, minced
2 medium tomatoes,
  peeled, seeded, and
  chopped

1/4 cup chicken broth
1/2 pound cooked
  crabmeat, shredded
1 tablespoon lemon juice
1/2 teaspoon celery salt
1/4 cup fresh parsley,
  chopped

Following package directions, cook the pasta in boiling water until *al dente*. Drain.

Melt the margarine or butter in a large skillet; sauté scallions and garlic until tender, about 3 minutes. Add the tomatoes and chicken broth; increase the heat and bring to a boil, stirring constantly. Reduce the heat and simmer for 2 minutes. Add the crabmeat, lemon juice, and celery salt. Cook until heated through, about 2 minutes. Stir in the chopped parsley.

Put the pasta on a serving dish. Top with the crabmeat mixture.

2 servings

&✿

PASTA WITH FENNEL

½ pound nonwheat
    linguine or angel hair
    pasta

2 teaspoons olive oil
2 cups of Fennel and
    Leeks (see page 101)

Cook the pasta to taste according to package directions. Drain.

Put the olive oil and 2 teaspoons of water in a medium skillet over medium heat. Stir in vegetables, cover, and cook until heated through.

Add the pasta and mix well.

2 servings

🕊

AVOCADO PASTA

At first, the idea of avocado with pasta didn't sound quite right to us. It seemed a bizarre combination. But it turned out to be so good that when we served it to our friend Leslie, her mood actually turned cheery, despite the fact that she'd just been given a $250 ticket for leaving her car momentarily in a handicapped parking space.

8 ounces nonwheat pasta	½ cup diced onion
¼ cup olive oil	4 garlic cloves, minced
1½ pounds tomatoes, seeded and diced	1 tablespoon chopped fresh parsley
3 ounces soy cheese, crumbled	1 tablespoon chopped fresh basil
1 large avocado, diced	

Following package directions, cook the pasta in boiling water until *al dente*. Drain.

Mix together the olive oil, tomatoes, cheese, avocado, onion, garlic, parsley, and basil in a large bowl.

Add the pasta and mix well.

4 servings

ᨾ

PASTA WITH SHRIMP

This is fine served cold at a picnic. People will think you bought it at the best local gourmet food mart.

Remember we were telling you about how salt makes a lot of these recipes taste better? Well, this is definitely one of them.

1 pound nonwheat pasta	1 teaspoon dried
1 pound medium shrimp,	oregano
shelled	2 small bunches arugula,
¼ cup plus 2 tablespoons	stemmed and
olive oil	chopped
2 shallots, chopped	1½ teaspoons lemon
8 sun-dried tomatoes	juice
packed in oil, cut into	
strips	

According to package directions, cook the pasta in boiling water until *al dente*. Drain.

Meanwhile, sauté the shrimp in 2 tablespoons of the olive oil in a medium skillet until pink, about 2 minutes.

Add the shallots, sun-dried tomatoes, and oregano. Cook, stirring occasionally, until shallots are soft, about 2 minutes. Scrape the mixture into a large bowl.

Add the arugula, ¼ cup of the olive oil, and the lemon juice. Stir well.

Add the pasta and mix well.

4 servings

PASTA WITH TOMATO AND GARLIC

The length of time you will need to simmer the tomatoes depends on their ripeness. Very ripe ones liquefy quickly when heated; less ripe ones hold their shape much longer. Since our taste is to have some tomato chunks with our pasta, we barely heat the tomatoes through before tossing with the pasta.

1 pound nonwheat pasta	12 plum tomatoes,
6 garlic cloves, minced	chopped
¼ cup olive oil	⅔ cup parsley, chopped

Cook pasta according to package directions. Drain.

Meanwhile, in a medium skillet, sauté the garlic in the oil over medium heat until soft, about 3 minutes. Add the tomatoes and parsley, lower heat, and simmer a short time. Toss pasta with sauce and serve.

4 servings

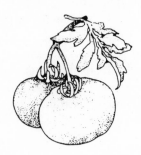

&.

CILANTRO CHICKEN WITH PASTA

To keep the chicken skin from sticking to the pan, dry chicken before sautéeing and keep heat moderate. If skin does stick, the chicken will still taste fine, but it may look as if somebody already ate it.

8 chicken legs
8 chicken thighs
1/2 cup olive oil
4 teaspoons cumin seed
1 teaspoon saffron threads
Juice of 2 lemons

3/4 cup fresh cilantro, chopped
4 cups chicken stock
2 cups small dried nonwheat pasta

Place chicken legs and thighs in a glass baking dish. In a bowl, combine the oil, cumin seed, saffron, lemon juice, and 1/2 cup of the cilantro. Pour over the chicken and turn to coat. Cover and marinate at room temperature for an hour or up to 4 hours in the refrigerator.

Heat two large, deep, heavy skillets over moderate heat. Pour 1/4 cup of the oil into each skillet and cook chicken, turning frequently until browned, about 15 minutes. Remove chicken to warmed plate and set aside.

Discard all the fat from the pans. Add 2 cups of stock to each pan and bring to a boil over high heat, scraping to dislodge any bits from the bottom. Pour all the stock into one pan, add the pasta, and cook for 4 minutes, stirring frequently.

Return the chicken to the pasta pan. Reduce heat, cover tightly, and simmer until the pasta and chicken are cooked thoroughly, about 20 minutes. Transfer chicken to plates and sprinkle remaining cilantro on top. Serve pasta alongside.

8 servings

Seafood

With fish, you can do a lot of substituting. Though a given recipe may call for swordfish, salmon would be fine, or shark, or halibut steaks. Buy what's on special and feel free to experiment.

See additional seafood recipes in chapter 6—Lunch.

🐟

MARINATED SWORDFISH WITH CILANTRO

Simple, elegant, easy, delicious. These are words more recipes would like to have said about them.

4 6-ounce swordfish (or   1 garlic clove, minced
   tuna or shark) steaks   3/4 cup fresh cilantro,
Juice of 2 limes   chopped
1/2 cup margarine or butter   Lime wedges

Put the fish in a glass baking dish. Pour the lime juice over. Marinate in the refrigerator for at least a half hour.

Melt the margarine or butter in a small saucepan. Add the garlic and cook for 30 seconds. Mix in the cilantro and cook until heated through, about 1 minute.

On a medium-hot grill, cook the fish until desired doneness, basting often with the cilantro margarine or butter. Serve fish with lime wedges.

4 servings

🙒

SWORDFISH WITH MINT AND LEMON

6 tablespoons unsalted
    margarine or butter,
    room temperature
4 teaspoons minced fresh
    mint
1 teaspoon grated lemon
    peel

4 6-ounce swordfish
    steaks
1/4 cup extra-virgin olive
    oil
Fresh mint leaves

Start grill or preheat broiler. Mix the margarine or butter, mint, and lemon peel in a small bowl. Shape the margarine or butter into a log, cover with wax paper, and refrigerate. (This can be made a day in advance.)

Put the fish in a shallow baking dish and drizzle with oil. Grill or broil fish until pink inside, about 4 minutes a side. Transfer the fish to plates, then top with a thick slice of mint-and-lemon margarine or butter. Garnish with mint leaves.

Note: The mint-and-lemon margarine or butter can be made in advance and kept up to a month in the freezer.

4 servings

🐦

SWORDFISH IN TOMATO AND FENNEL SAUCE

That licoricy fennel taste pervades this, thanks to the fennel seeds. You might want to give them a couple of bashes in a mortar and pestle before throwing them in, to release even more flavor.

2 tablespoons olive oil
1 small fennel bulb,
    trimmed, quartered,
    and sliced crosswise
    (can substitute 2 celery
    stalks, sliced 1/4-inch
    thick)
1/2 cup onion, chopped
1 garlic clove, minced
1/2 teaspoon fennel seeds

1 orange peel strip,
    diced
3 lemon peel strips,
    diced
1 16-ounce can Italian
    plum tomatoes,
    undrained
4 swordfish steaks
4 thin lemon slices

Heat oil in a stovetop-to-oven baking dish over medium-low heat. Add fennel and onion and sauté until tender, about 10 minutes. Stir in garlic and sauté 1 minute. Add fennel seeds, orange and lemon peels, and tomatoes with liquid. Bring to boil over low heat, stirring constantly, breaking up tomatoes with spoon. Simmer sauce until reduced slightly, about 10 minutes.

    Preheat broiler. Arrange fish on top of the tomato mixture. Broil 2 inches from heat until fish is opaque, about 5 minutes.

    Serve fish on heated plates. Spoon on sauce. Garnish with lemon slices and reserved fennel tops.

4 servings

❧

SWORDFISH AND SALSA

This is great grilled, too. And really easy—your guests think they're getting something you slaved over, but it takes less than half an hour.

4 swordfish steaks	Simple Salsa (see page
4 tablespoons margarine or	160)
butter, melted	

Preheat broiler and arrange fish on a broiling rack. Brush each steak with ½ tablespoon of the melted margarine or butter. Broil fish 4 inches from heat for about 4 minutes. Turn steaks over and brush each with ½ tablespoon of margarine or butter. Broil 4 minutes longer, until fish is opaque. Transfer to a warm plate and top with salsa.

4 servings

❧

GRILLED SHARK WITH TOMATOES
AND HERBS

3 tomatoes, peeled, seeded, and chopped

1/2 cup extra-virgin olive oil

3 tablespoons lemon juice

3 garlic cloves, minced

2 tablespoons chopped chervil

2 tablespoons chopped chives

2 tablespoons chopped tarragon

4 shark (or tuna or swordfish) steaks

In a medium bowl, blend together tomatoes, olive oil, lemon juice, and garlic. Add the fish, and set aside for 2 hours. Then add all the herbs, mixing well.

Grill the fish on a preheated broiler 4 inches from the heat, turning once, until charred on the outside, about 3 to 4 minutes on each side.

When the fish is done, transfer it onto a large platter and cut it into thick strips. Top with half of the tomato sauce and put the rest of the sauce in a bowl to pass.

4 servings

❧

SALMON WITH LIME

This is an extremely quick and easy recipe. But to make it even easier on yourself, have the butcher make those paper-thin slices for you. We could be saving you a fingertip here, too.
This defines that now familiar litany: easy, quick, delicious.

1 pound salmon fillets	Juice of half a lime
2 shallots, chopped	Lime peel, grated
4 tablespoons margarine or butter	

Heat oven to 350 degrees F. Put four ovenproof plates in preheated oven to warm, about 3 minutes. Then cut salmon into paper-thin slices.

Sauté chopped shallots in margarine or butter until slightly brown. Squeeze in lime juice and sprinkle in peel. Stir. When margarine or butter sizzles, coat each plate with 1/2 tablespoon of margarine or butter and immediately put fish on hot plates. Pour remaining butter over salmon and serve immediately.

4 servings

❧

GRILLED TUNA AND EGGPLANT

¹/₄ cup olive oil
1 1-pound eggplant, cut
    into ¹/₄-inch-thick slices
1 sweet red pepper

¹/₂ teaspoon rosemary,
    crumbled
1 pound tuna steak

Preheat broiler.

Heat 2 tablespoons of the olive oil in a large skillet over medium-high heat. Add the eggplant and cook until browned on both sides, adding more oil if necessary. Remove from the heat and set aside.

Broil the red pepper about 10 minutes, or until all sides are blistered. Put the pepper in a paper bag and let stand 10 minutes. Under cold water, gently rub the pepper to peel off the skin. Remove the seeds and slice the pepper.

If desired, chop the eggplant, then combine the eggplant and red pepper with 2 tablespoons of the olive oil and rosemary. Let stand for 30 minutes.

Grill or broil tuna for about 1 to 3 minutes per side until medium rare. Place the tuna on a serving plate and cover with the eggplant mixture.

4 servings

SHRIMP CREOLE

1 tablespoon margarine or butter	1 bay leaf
2 cups onion, finely chopped	2 sprigs fresh thyme or 1 teaspoon dried
2 cups celery, minced	6 cups canned chopped tomatoes
1 cup green pepper, minced	2 teaspoons curry powder
1 garlic clove, minced	2 pounds raw shrimp, shelled and deveined
1 teaspoon fennel seeds	
½ cup parsley, minced	

Heat margarine or butter in a medium saucepan. Add onion, celery, green pepper, garlic, and fennel seeds. Cook, stirring, until onion is tender, about 5 minutes.

Add remaining ingredients except for shrimp. Bring to a boil and simmer 15 minutes, stirring occasionally.

Add shrimp and cook until done, 5 to 10 minutes more.

6 servings

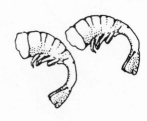

❧

SCALLOPS IN HERBS

The fresh herbs really make this one sing. Serve it in custard cups as a first course, or with rice and a green salad as a main course. Either way, the tarragon is the key. As James Brown once said, "Ow!"

6 tablespoons margarine or butter

4 shallots, peeled and chopped

2 garlic cloves, chopped

2 pounds bay scallops

2 tablespoons chopped parsley

1 tablespoon chopped chives

1 tablespoon chopped tarragon

Melt the margarine or butter in a sauté pan, add the shallots and garlic, and sauté until tender, about 2 minutes. Then add the scallops and herbs, and sauté until the scallops are cooked, another minute or two.

If you want, you can put a quarter pound of scallops each in custard cups, pour the sautéed shallots and garlic on top, and sprinkle the herbs on top. Then bake at 425 degrees F. for about 10 minutes and serve the herbed scallops in the cups.

4 servings as an entrée, 8 as a first course

❧

RICE PILAF WITH SHRIMP

3 tablespoons olive oil
1 pound medium shrimp,
    shelled and deveined
2 small zucchini, cut into
    thin sticks
1/2 cup onion, minced
1 garlic clove, minced

1 1/4 cups long-grain rice
2 1/2 cups hot water
1/2 teaspoon dried
    thyme, crumbled
1 bay leaf
2 tablespoons cilantro,
    minced

Heat 2 tablespoons of the oil in a sauté pan. Add the shrimp and sauté for 2 minutes. Remove shrimp. Add the zucchini and sauté for 2 minutes. Remove zucchini.

Add the remaining tablespoon of oil to the pan along with the onion. Sauté over medium heat until tender, but not brown, about 7 minutes. Add garlic and rice and sauté another 3 minutes.

Pour the hot water over the rice and stir. Add the thyme and the bay leaf. Bring to a boil over high heat. Then lower heat, cover, and simmer for 25 to 30 minutes until liquid is absorbed. Scatter the shrimp and zucchini over the top. Simmer, covered, for an additional 3 to 5 minutes until rice is tender. Discard the bay leaf.

Top with the cilantro. Serve.

4 servings

Birds

Here we are referring not to Charlie Parker and Larry Byrd, but to those small, wing-flapping, squawking things that taste so good with tarragon. Chicken, cornish hen, and turkey. But increasingly pheasant, quail, and other formerly exotic, hard-to-find avians are becoming available.

Standard roast recipes can be found in other cookbooks. So let's get on with some others here.

?♣

CHICKEN PROVENÇAL

2 chicken breast halves,
  skinned and boned
1 tablespoon olive oil
4 tablespoons margarine or
  butter
4 ounces soy cheese

2 small tomatoes, sliced
1 tablespoon chopped
  fresh rosemary or 3/4
  teaspoon dried
1/2 cup chicken broth

Place the breast halves between sheets of wax paper. Pound with a meat hammer until flattened.

Over medium-high heat, heat oil and 2 tablespoons margarine or butter in a large skillet. Sauté breasts until golden on both sides. Arrange alternating slices of cheese and tomato on each breast, and sprinkle with rosemary. Pour broth over chicken and cover.

Lower heat and cook for about 3 minutes, until cheese and tomato are warmed through. Cheese should not melt completely. Remove chicken to warm platter. Over high heat, boil sauce rapidly down. Slowly stir in the remaining margarine or butter, a tablespoon at a time. Pour sauce over chicken.

4 servings

❧

GRILLED MARINATED CHICKEN BREASTS

Perfect grill food, with flavor intensity. Start preparing it at least 4 hours before you want to serve it. A major crowd-pleaser.

³/4 cup lemon juice	1¹/2 teaspoons thyme
³/4 cup vegetable oil	12 chicken breast halves,
¹/4 cup minced onion	skinned and boned

In a medium bowl, mix together the lemon juice, oil, onion, and thyme. With a sharp knife, make small cuts in each chicken breast. Pour one-third of the marinade into a shallow glass bowl or baking dish. Add half the chicken and cover with one-third of the marinade. Layer the remaining chicken on top and add the remaining marinade. Let stand in the refrigerator for 3 hours, turning occasionally. Remove from the refrigerator for an hour to bring to room temperature.

Cook chicken on a grill or under a preheated broiler, 3 minutes or more per side. Do not overcook, as breasts will become dry and chewy. To check for doneness, slice into a breast — it should be *slightly* pink at the center.

6 servings

❧

MIXED GRILL

We make this all the time, and always love it—it's got legs, literally and figuratively. That's because the chicken and shrimp, following their marination, are imbued with all these delicious flavors. You co-diners not on the diet could precook a couple of sausages in a pan of boiling water, then add chunks to the skewers. They bring in a nice third flavor.

1/2 cup olive oil	8 large shrimp
2 garlic cloves, minced	1 red onion, cut in
1 teaspoon dried sage	chunks
1/2 teaspoon dried thyme	
2 tablespoons lemon juice	
2 chicken thighs, boned, skinned, and cut into 4 pieces each	

Mix the olive oil, garlic, sage, thyme, and lemon juice in a glass bowl. Add the chicken and shrimp and stir. Let stand for 20 minutes.

Heat the grill or broiler.

Drain chicken and shrimp, reserving marinade. Alternating chicken, shrimp, and onion pieces, thread onto skewers. Cook, turning the skewers and basting with marinade, until the meat is done, 10 to 15 minutes.

4 servings

🍮

SOUTH OF THE BORDER MILLET AND CHICKEN IN LETTUCE

An off-the-beaten-path sort of dinner, and perfect in hot weather.

1 cup millet
1/4 cup lime juice (about 2 limes)
2 tablespoons olive oil
1 garlic clove, pressed
4 scallions, chopped
1/2 cup chopped red bell pepper
2 tablespoons minced fresh cilantro

1 cup cooked chicken or turkey, chopped
1 cup chopped tomato
1 cup cilantro, chopped
1 avocado, peeled and sliced
12 large lettuce leaves

Cook the millet in a large pot of boiling water for 20 minutes. Drain and fluff the millet with a fork. Allow to cool.

Whisk the lime juice, olive oil, and garlic in a large bowl. Add the cooked millet, scallions, bell pepper, and minced cilantro, and toss.

Put the chicken or turkey, chopped tomatoes, chopped cilantro, and sliced avocado on individual serving plates. Arrange lettuce leaves on a platter. Station these pleasingly around the dinner table.

Give everyone a good helping of the millet mixture. Pass the lettuce leaves, then the other ingredients.

4 servings

🕊

ROSEMARY CHICKEN BREASTS
WITH SHALLOT

1 shallot
6 tablespoons softened
   margarine or butter
1/2 tablespoon fresh ground
   pepper
Fresh lemon juice

4 large chicken breasts,
   bone removed
1 tablespoon oil
2 tablespoons minced
   fresh rosemary

Mince shallot. Beat into margarine or butter; add pepper. Season to taste with lemon juice. Roll into a 1-inch log, wrap in plastic, and refrigerate.

Rub breasts with oil and rosemary. Grill or broil chicken, turning once, until done — about 10 minutes. Top each breast with a quarter-inch slice of margarine or butter and serve.

4 servings

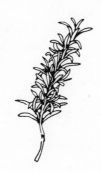

🐌

MICROWAVE CHICKEN

2 tablespoons olive oil	2 teaspoons paprika
1 chicken, disjointed, breasts halved	1/2 teaspoon fennel seeds
1 onion, minced	1/2 teaspoon ground coriander
1 red pepper, cored, seeded, and minced	1 1/2 cups frozen peas
1 garlic clove, minced	2 tablespoons water
1 cup rice, cooked	2 tablespoons minced cilantro
1 12-ounce can chopped tomatoes with juice	

Heat oil in a large, heavy skillet. Add chicken and brown on all sides, about 5 minutes. Transfer to a platter and set aside.

Sauté onion, pepper, and garlic in drippings for 2 minutes. Transfer to a 5-quart microwave casserole.

Stir rice, tomatoes, paprika, fennel, and ground coriander into the casserole. Arrange chicken on top, largest pieces toward the outside, wings in the center.

Cover and microwave on high for 12 minutes. Turn chicken over, stir rice, and rotate dish 180 degrees. Microwave an additional 12 minutes or until chicken is done and rice is tender. (Remember, every microwave is different; some will require more or less cooking time.) Let stand, covered, a few minutes.

Meanwhile, microwave peas with water in covered 1-pint casserole on high for 5 minutes, stirring at 2 minutes. Cook until tender. Drain well. Stir into chicken-and-rice mixture. Sprinkle with cilantro and serve.

6 servings

🍂

CHICKEN AND CILANTRO

A perfect midweek throw-together dinner. Just make some rice to go with it. The cilantro gives it a nice flavor intensity.

2½ tablespoons oil
2 small green peppers,
    sliced in rings
1½ pounds skinless,
    boneless chicken thighs
2 8-ounce cans of tomato
    sauce or 16 ounces of
    fresh Tomato Sauce
    (see page 156)

1 cup cilantro, chopped
½ cup chopped onion
1 garlic clove, minced

Heat 1 tablespoon of oil in skillet; add pepper rings, and fry until soft, about 15 minutes. Drain on absorbent towels. Add the remaining oil and the chicken and sauté until done, about 25 to 30 minutes.

Meanwhile, put the tomato sauce, cilantro, onion, and garlic into a blender. Blend well. Pour entire mixture over the chicken. When contents of pan boil, reduce heat, cover, and simmer for 5 minutes. When chicken is tender, serve with pepper rings on top.

6 servings

&.

CHICKEN AND SQUASH WITH HERBS

It's the tarragon and the nicely crisped chicken skin that make this dish special. If you're just making two servings, use your toaster oven.

Herb margarine or butter:

1/4 pound margarine or
butter, softened

2 garlic cloves, minced

1/2 cup fresh basil,
tarragon, or parsley,
chopped

4 whole chicken legs

2 yellow squash, cut in
1/4-inch slices

2 zucchini, cut in
1/4-inch slices

Mix the margarine or butter, garlic, and herbs together. Refrigerate if desired.

Preheat the oven to 425 degrees F. Dot the chicken under the skin with 4 tablespoons of the herb margarine or butter. Bake in an uncovered casserole for 35 minutes.

Just before chicken is done, heat the rest of the herb margarine or butter in a large pan. Add squash and zucchini and sauté until tender, a few minutes at most. Serve the chicken surrounded by the squash.

Note: The herb margarine or butter can be kept up to a month in the freezer.

4 servings

❧

CHICKEN AND FRESH HERB PESTO

4 scallions, cut into 1/2-inch
  pieces
4 large garlic cloves
1/2 cup fresh Italian parsley
  leaves
1/4 cup fresh tarragon or
  basil leaves

2 tablespoons of walnut
  pieces or pine nuts
1 1/2 teaspoons of grated
  lemon peel
1/3 cup olive oil
4 whole chicken legs

Preheat the oven to 450 degrees F.

Put scallions, garlic, parsley, tarragon or basil, nuts, and lemon peel into a food processor. While the machine is running, add oil slowly until the mixture is a coarse paste.

Grease a medium-size casserole. Put in chicken and spread with pesto. Bake until tender, about 40 minutes. Baste only once.

4 servings

❧

BAKED CHICKEN WITH ROOT VEGETABLES

2 large carrots, peeled and
cut in 1-inch pieces
2 parsnips, peeled and cut
in 1-inch pieces
1 rutabaga, peeled and cut
in 1-inch pieces
1 medium onion, quartered

2 tablespoons plus 2
teaspoons of olive oil
1 teaspoon sage
1 teaspoon dried
rosemary
2 whole chicken legs
2 garlic cloves, crushed

Preheat the oven to 375 degrees F. Put the carrots, parsnips, rutabaga, and onion in a medium-size baking pan. Add 2 tablespoons of the oil, 1/2 teaspoon of the sage, and 1/2 teaspoon of the rosemary. Stir all ingredients. Bake, covered, for 30 minutes.

Meanwhile, rub the chicken with garlic, then with the remaining 2 teaspoons of oil and the remaining 1/2 teaspoons of the sage and rosemary. Add the chicken to the vegetables. Cook an additional hour, stirring the vegetables occasionally.

2 servings

❧

CHICKEN À LA CHRIS

Your basic chicken sauté, and a tasty little sucker at that. If you want a treat sometime, try deglazing the pan with white wine instead of chicken broth.

4 chicken breast halves,
    skinned
1 tablespoon olive oil
2 garlic cloves, minced
1 medium onion, chopped
1 red pepper, cut in strips

1 green pepper, cut in
    strips
1½ cups chicken broth
¼ cup tomato paste
1 tablespoon minced
    cilantro

Sauté the chicken in the olive oil in a large pan until lightly browned on both sides. Remove the chicken. Add the garlic, onion, and peppers, and cook for approximately 2 minutes. Add the chicken broth and tomato paste. Simmer, covered, 5 minutes. Return chicken to pan and simmer, uncovered, another 10 minutes. Stir in cilantro and serve.

4 servings

ﹸ

GRILLED TURKEY BROCHETTE

An old favorite around our house. The usual adjectives—quick, easy, delicious...

6 tablespoons lemon juice
1 tablespoon sesame oil
8 ounces turkey breast, cut
   in 1½-inch cubes
1 small zucchini, cut in
   chunks

1 red pepper, cored,
   seeded, and cut up
1 purple onion, peeled
   and cut in chunks

Combine lemon juice and oil in a small bowl. Add turkey cubes and marinate in refrigerator for at least an hour.

Thread turkey chunks onto skewers, alternating with vegetables. Grill 15 minutes, turning several times and basting with marinade.

2 servings

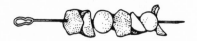

ROAST CHICKEN WITH GARLIC

Nothing like a good, old-fashioned roast chicken. This one's particularly succulent.

1 3-to-4 pound chicken	2 tablespoons olive oil
10 large garlic cloves	3 tablespoons chicken
1 tablespoon dried oregano	broth

Preheat oven to 450 degrees F.

Rinse chicken and pat dry. Place breast side up in foil-lined roasting pan. Split 8 garlic cloves and put them, along with ½ tablespoon of the oregano, into the chicken cavity.

Mince the remaining garlic. Mix with the remaining oregano, oil, and broth. Carefully separate skin from breast meat of chicken, making a pocket. Spoon half of the garlic mixture into the pocket and distribute evenly.

Smear remaining garlic mixture over the surface of the chicken. Tuck wings under chicken body and place in center of oven. Roast until juices from thigh have turned from rosy to clear, about 50 minutes. Let chicken rest 10 minutes; then carve and serve.

4 servings

🐚

TURKEY THIGHS WITH VEGETABLE SAUCE

1 1/2 cups chicken broth
3 pounds turkey thighs
1 1/2 tablespoons oil or
    melted margarine or
    butter
1 1/2 teaspoons oregano
1/4 cup olive oil
1 onion, sliced
2 patty pan squash, sliced

2 yellow crookneck
    squash, sliced
1 bunch radishes, cut in
    halves
Juice of 1 lemon
2 tomatoes, diced
2 tablespoons chopped
    fresh basil

Pour 1 cup of the chicken broth into a shallow baking dish. Rub turkey thighs lightly with the oil. Sprinkle with the oregano and place in the baking dish. Bake at 325 degrees F. for an hour, basting occasionally.

Heat the olive oil in a skillet and sauté the onion until tender. Stir in the patty pan squash, yellow squash, and radishes. Sauté 3 minutes. Add remaining broth and lemon juice. Simmer until vegetables are tender-crisp. Add tomatoes and basil, and stir until heated through.

Serve thighs with the vegetables on the side.

4 servings

Meat

Many of us had a sneaking suspicion that eating a lot of meat, especially red meat, might not be all that good for us. Now there is scientific evidence to support that. In fact, current research suggests that meat can actually depress our immune systems. But we don't let that keep us from enjoying meat on occasion. It's another of those "in moderation" propositions. The following recipes are delicious and fun—just don't get in the habit of eating meat every night.

❧

LAMB CHOPS WITH GARLIC AND ROSEMARY

As classic and elegant as a tuxedo. Ahhhhh.

1 or 2 3-inch-thick loin
    lamb chops per person,
    depending on appetite

Fresh rosemary
2 garlic cloves, sliced
Olive oil

Preheat broiler.

Rub chops with rosemary and garlic. Poke slits with point of knife, six on each side of chop. Insert little bunches of rosemary needles in the slits on top, and thin slices of garlic in the ones on the bottom.

Tie chops around the perimeter with cotton string to prevent "tail" from drying. Rub with olive oil. Place 4 inches under heat in broiler. Broil 5 minutes per side, then begin checking for desired degree of doneness.

☙

LAMB CHOPS WITH TOMATO

4 tablespoons softened
   margarine or butter
1½ whole sun-dried
   tomatoes
2 tablespoons minced
   parsley

1 or 2 1-inch-thick
   shoulder lamb chops
   per person

Cream margarine or butter and tomatoes by hand or in a food processor. Put mixture in wax paper and roll into a log. Chill at least an hour in the refrigerator.

Heat broiler. Broil chops 4 minutes per side until done. Sprinkle with parsley and top with a slice of margarine or butter.

Note: Tomato-margarine or -butter can be kept up to a month in the freezer.

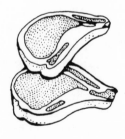

🍃

GREEK LAMB

Even before there was CFS in our house, this was the one we cooked for guests when we were tired. No browning or anything—just toss the meat and other ingredients in your pan and bake. It comes out great every time.

You should get your butcher to do the cubing of the meat, as that is time consuming.

3½ pounds lamb shoulder, cut in 1-inch cubes
2 garlic cloves
⅔ cup tomato paste (beware of sugar)
1 large onion, chopped
1 teaspoon basil

½ cup celery leaves, chopped
½ teaspoon dried oregano
½ cup dill, chopped
1 cup parsley, chopped

Preheat the oven to 350 degrees F. Put lamb into a large pan. Top with all other ingredients except half of the basil and parsley. Toss to mix. Cover and bake for an hour.

Reduce oven to 300 degrees F. and bake for another 30 minutes, until the meat is tender. Sprinkle with the remaining herbs and serve.

8 servings

🕹

SKILLET LAMB WITH EGGPLANT

3 tablespoons olive oil
2 pounds of boneless lamb,
    shoulder or leg, cubed
2 large onions, sliced
1 eggplant, peeled and
    chopped

$^1/_4$ cup tomato purée
1 cup chicken stock
1 tomato, diced
Chopped parsley

Heat the oil in a large frying pan; add the meat and onions
and cook until onions are tender and meat is browned.

Add the eggplant to the lamb and brown lightly. Mix in
the tomato purée and chicken stock. Cover and simmer for 45
minutes.

Serve, sprinkling each portion with tomato and parsley.

4 servings

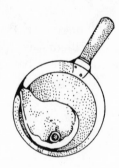

≈

MEATBALLS WITH KALE

This recipe is delicious in an earthy, real-world sort of way—which is the way we like it. It is, however, somewhat labor intensive, so this isn't one to take on if you're having a tired day. The workload can be made less onerous by making the meatballs earlier and keeping them in the fridge until you're ready to cook them.

1/2 cup barley
1 tablespoon margarine or
   butter
3/4 pound kale leaves, stems
   removed, chopped
1 1/4 cups chicken broth
1 1/2 pounds ground lamb
1 medium onion, minced

3 tablespoons fine-
   chopped parsley
1 egg, beaten
1/8 teaspoon nutmeg
2 teaspoons olive oil
2 garlic cloves, crushed
1 teaspoon ground
   coriander

Cook the barley in a large pot of boiling water, partially covered, for 20 minutes. Drain and set aside.

At the same time, melt the margarine or butter in a large pot. Add the kale and 1/2 cup of the chicken broth. Simmer for 20 minutes, covered.

Meanwhile, mix lamb, onion, parsley, egg, remaining 1/4 cup of the chicken broth, and nutmeg in a large bowl. Stir well and shape into balls. If onion is not chopped fine enough, the balls will not hold together well.

Rub a heavy skillet with 1 teaspoon of the olive oil. Sauté the meatballs, a batch at a time, over medium-high heat, until lightly browned on all sides.

Mash the garlic and coriander into a paste. Heat the remaining teaspoon of olive oil in a small pan over medium heat. Add the garlic mixture and sauté for about 3 minutes.

Drain excess liquid from the kale, then stir in the garlic mixture. Add the barley, meatballs, and remaining half cup of chicken broth and mix well. Simmer, covered, for 30 minutes, adding more chicken broth or water if necessary.

6 servings

🕏

MEATBALL SHISH KEBABS

More grill-driven, back-porch food. It's great—what's not to like?

1½ pounds ground lamb
1 teaspoon dried mint
½ cup chopped parsley
2 garlic cloves, minced
16 1-inch chunks red onion
16 cherry tomatoes
16 1-inch cubes green bell pepper

Put the lamb, mint, parsley, and garlic in a medium-size bowl. Stir well. Shape the meat into 14 to 16 1-inch balls. Balls must be firm to prevent them from falling off the skewers while cooking.

Place the meatballs onto skewers, alternating with onion chunks, tomatoes, and pepper pieces. Put the skewers into the refrigerator until ready to grill.

Cook over medium-hot coals, or on cooktop grill, turning every 3 or 4 minutes until the meat is done — about 15 minutes in all.

6 servings

🐇

MARINATED GRILLED RABBIT

1 cup vegetable oil	$1/2$ teaspoon garlic salt
2 tablespoons lemon juice	1 rabbit, about 3
1 teaspoon lemon peel,	pounds, cut in 6
grated	pieces
1 teaspoon paprika	1 tablespoon minced
2 teaspoons fresh thyme	parsley

Mix the oil, lemon juice, lemon peel, paprika, thyme, and garlic salt in a pan just big enough to hold all the rabbit pieces. Refrigerate the rabbit in the marinade for an hour, turning every 15 minutes.

Remove the rabbit from the marinade; grill slowly for 30 minutes. Use the remaining marinade for basting. When the rabbit is done, serve on warm plates, pouring the remaining marinade over the rabbit.

6 servings

∽ 8 ∾

Sauces, Ingredients, and Accompaniments

Here are the adjusted versions of many of the sauces and other foods you took for granted. Also, some accompaniments to make eating more interesting, and even some dipping concoctions for corn chips while you're watching TV.

🐚

TOMATO SAUCE

Here's a good place to take advantage of the cans of already chopped, peeled tomatoes available these days in supermarkets. Why work if they're going to do it for you?

3 cups canned tomatoes, chopped, most of the juice discarded

1/2 teaspoon garlic powder

1/4 teaspoon rosemary, minced

2 tablespoons water

Combine tomatoes, garlic powder, rosemary, and water in a small saucepan. Bring to a boil.

Reduce heat and simmer, covered, stirring occasionally, until tomatoes are softened, about 4 minutes.

Serve warm or cold with almost anything.

3 cups

❧

MAYONNAISE

2 eggs   1¹/₂ cups light olive oil
1 tablespoon lemon juice

Put eggs and lemon juice in a blender or food processer and mix on high for 5 seconds. While machine is still running, slowly add oil in a steady stream. As it thickens, add the remaining oil quickly. Stop blender when mayonnaise is thick.

About 2 cups

❧

"VINAIGRETTE"

All right, it's not true vinaigrette. We're lying. But if you can't have vinegar right now, this'll do. Think of it as "lemonaigrette." It's pretty good. Use a good, flavorful olive oil, and you'll like this fine.

2 tablespoons lemon juice   8 tablespoons olive oil

In a small bowl mix lemon juice and olive oil. Taste it, and then add either more lemon juice or more olive oil according to taste.

Note: You may add minced garlic, shallots, onions, or any herb you might have handy to this basic recipe for an additional flavor element.

²/₃ cup

❧

TAHINI SAUCE

Tahini is made entirely of sesame seeds. The sauce is wonderful as a dip, on rice cakes, or to spice up fish or chicken.

3/4 cup Tahini (can be found in most health food stores and some supermarkets)

Juice of 3 or 4 lemons
1/2 teaspoon garlic powder

Combine all ingredients and mix well. If sauce is too thick, add water until mixture reaches proper consistency.

1 cup

🖈

PEPPER-AVOCADO SALSA

This is a great dip with corn chips, or to serve with chicken, fish, or even meat. If you're feeling tired, don't bother roasting and peeling the peppers—it's an annoying task.

2 tablespoons olive oil
1/2 cup chopped onions
2 garlic cloves, chopped
1 pound tomatillos, peeled
    and quartered
1 pound plum tomatoes,
    quartered
1/2 teaspoon ground cumin
1 red bell pepper, roasted,
    peeled, and seeded

1 green bell pepper,
    roasted, peeled, and
    seeded
1/2 avocado, chopped
1 tablespoon chopped
    cilantro

Put olive oil in large pan over medium heat. Add onions, garlic, tomatillos, tomatoes, and cumin, and cook for 20 minutes. Add peppers and place the mixture in a food processor or blender and blend coarsely with on-off pulses. Bring to room temperature; mix in the avocado and cilantro.

2 quarts

₰

SIMPLE SALSA

For a different flavor, try adding chopped tomatoes. This salsa will keep about a week in the refrigerator.

1 ripe avocado, chopped
 into 1/4-inch pieces
3 tablespoons olive oil
2 1/2 tablespoons lime juice
1/3 cup scallions, chopped

1 garlic clove, crushed
2 tablespoons chopped
 fresh cilantro

In a medium bowl, combine all ingredients. Stir well.

2 cups

₰

HOLLANDAISE SAUCE

It's nice that a luxurious item like this is 100 percent okay for this diet. If it doesn't emulsify with margarine, use butter. Have it on vegetables, eggs Benedict, and so forth.

1/4 cup margarine or butter
2 egg yolks

2 teaspoons lemon juice

Melt margarine or butter in saucepan. Mix egg yolks and lemon juice in a blender, at low speed. Remove the cover and continue to blend, while adding the margarine or butter in a steady, narrow stream. Hollandaise will thicken. When all the margarine or butter has been added, the sauce is ready to serve.

3/4 cup

✺

MARINARA SAUCE

1½ cups onion, chopped
1 carrot, diced
3 tablespoons olive oil
4 garlic cloves, crushed
1 28-ounce can tomato
　　purée

3 tablespoons chopped
　　fresh basil
1 teaspoon dried
　　oregano

Sauté the onions and carrot in olive oil until onions are tender.
When almost finished, add the garlic. Then add the tomato
purée, basil, and oregano. Cook over low-medium heat until
thickened, about 20 minutes.

Makes 3 cups

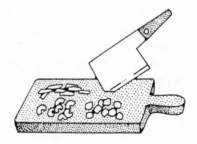

&.

MICROWAVE CHICKEN STOCK

Oven cooking bags may burst during microwave cooking. Read the package directions carefully to learn how to avoid this.

1 onion, quartered	1 chicken, about 3
2 celery stalks, quartered	pounds
1 medium carrot, quartered	Oven cooking bag
1 bay leaf	
1 thyme sprig	

Stuff chicken with as much of the other ingredients as you can fit into the cavity. Put the stuffed chicken in an oven cooking bag, and put the bag in a large, microwave-safe bowl. Add 3 cups of water to the bag and tie a loose knot to close it.

Microwave on high for 20 minutes, more if the chicken weighs more than 3 pounds. Turn over halfway through cooking. Reduce power to defrost and cook another fifteen minutes. Strain stock; remove and discard the vegetables. Save poached chicken to make chicken salad.

Note: Times should be increased by 50 percent for smaller ovens.

3 cups

PART THREE

The Phase Two Diet

The Phase Two Diet

Congratulations! You've worked hard to eat the right foods, and you should be feeling much better and stronger. Now the time has come for a little variation—to find out what your body can tolerate and what it can't. Here are a few recipes to get you started. Try them, and don't forget to experiment with some of your own.

Remember to reintroduce new foods one at a time and gauge your response to each one. If a given food creates a problem, discontinue it.

∾ 9 ∽

Breakfast

Even now you must be careful about cereal. Maybe only one in fifty is made without sugar. Puffed wheat, corn, and millet cereals can be found that contain nothing but wheat, corn, or millet. It's worth the search—they taste good with milk substitutes and fruit. (For suggestions on some allowable cereals, see our list in part 1, chapter 3.)

If you find you can now tolerate fruit, it makes a nice breakfast all by itself. Cantaloupe with lime is a major treat. Mango for breakfast is close to sin. The one caveat—you'll probably run out of fuel halfway through the morning, so have some nuts or other snacks on hand when the munchies strike.

Also remember that fresh-juiced fruit is delicious. Juiced honeydew with lime, for instance, is awesome. Experiment with your own mixtures. Remember, though, it must be *fresh*, either juiced yourself or at a health food store or juice bar. V-8 and the like won't do. In many commercially prepared juices, the naturally occurring enzymes have broken down and lost their nutritional value.

❧

"STANDARD" BREAKFAST

This is an ultra-easy breakfast that never gets boring. We have it almost every day.

½ cup corn cereal (can be bought at health food stores and some supermarkets)

¼ cup milk substitute
½ banana, sliced

Pour cereal into a bowl, top with milk, and add bananas.

1 serving

❧

BREAKFAST COUSCOUS

2 cups water
¼ teaspoon cinnamon

1 cup instant couscous
Margarine or butter

In a medium-size saucepan, combine the water and cinnamon and bring to a boil. Pour in the couscous, reduce the heat to a simmer, and cook for 30 seconds.

Remove from heat, cover, and let stand for at least 5 minutes, until the liquid is absorbed. Top with butter and serve.

2 servings

🐌

CRANBERRY TUMBLER

¹/₂ cup unsweetened
    cranberry juice
¹/₂ cup seltzer

¹/₂ teaspoon lemon juice
Sprig of mint

Mix together in a glass.

1 serving

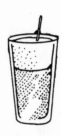

~ 10 ~

Lunch

❧

TABBOULEH

½ cup bulgur wheat
1 cup boiling water
1½ cups fresh parsley,
    chopped
4 scallions, chopped

1 large tomato, chopped
6 sprigs mint, chopped
Juice of 1½ lemons
¼ cup olive oil

Pour boiling water over bulgur wheat. Let stand for an hour. In a large bowl, mix parsley, scallions, tomato, mint, and bulgur wheat. Add the lemon juice and olive oil and mix well.

4 servings

❧

SPECIAL QUESADILLAS

⅔ cup corn kernels
1 teaspoon water
2 large scallions, sliced thin
2 tablespoons cilantro
    leaves
2 teaspoons oil

4 flour tortillas
8 ounces soy cheese,
    sliced thin
Simple Salsa (see page
    160)

Combine corn, water, scallions, and cilantro leaves in a small bowl. Heat half the oil in a large skillet. Place a tortilla in the skillet, and cover it with a layer of cheese. Top with some of the corn mixture, and layer on more cheese. Top with another tortilla and cook approximately 3 minutes on each side.

Repeat for second quesadilla. Cut quesadillas into wedges. Serve with salsa.

2 servings

🐟

SPECIAL BURGERS

A sort of Middle Eastern thing, with bold flavors and a nice crunchy texture. With ketchup, it's an easy sell to kids.

³/4 cup boiling water
¹/4 cup bulgur wheat
¹/3 cup whole natural
   almonds
1 pound lean ground
   turkey

¹/4 cup vegetable oil
¹/4 cup chopped red
   onion
1 teaspoon garlic salt
1 teaspoon dried basil

Preheat oven to 350 degrees F. Pour water over the bulgur and let stand until cool.

Put the almonds in a single layer on a baking sheet. Bake for 15 minutes, stirring occasionally, until lightly toasted. Cool, then chop.

Drain bulgur well. Then add the almonds, turkey, oil, red onion, garlic salt, and basil, and mix well. Shape into 6 patties. Grill, broil, or sauté until meat is done to your taste.

6 servings

❧

GREEK BURGERS

¹/₄ cup vegetable oil
1¹/₂ pounds ground turkey
¹/₄ cup scallions, chopped
1 teaspoon dried oregano
    leaves, crumbled

¹/₂ teaspoon garlic
    powder
2 ounces soy cheese,
    crumbled
Juice of 1 lemon

Add oil to ground turkey; mix well. Add the remaining ingredients and mix well.

Fry or grill patties, about 6 minutes per side, until meat reaches desired doneness.

6 servings

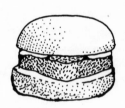

✺ 11 ✺

Dinner

✺

COUSCOUS WITH SAGE

A nicely different way to put a grain on the plate.

1/2 cup chicken broth
1/2 teaspoon crumbled
dried sage
1/2 cup couscous

2 teaspoons unsalted
margarine or butter,
cut in pieces

In a small saucepan boil chicken broth and sage; stir in couscous and remove from heat. Let the couscous stand, covered, for 5 minutes, then add the margarine or butter. Fluff with a fork and serve.

2 servings

❧

PILAF WITH CASHEWS

1 medium onion, sliced
thin
1 tablespoon margarine or
butter
½ cup bulgur wheat
¾ cup chicken broth

3 tablespoons chopped
dry-roasted, unsalted
cashews
1 tablespoon chopped
scallions

In a small saucepan, cook onion in margarine or butter until tender. Add bulgur and cook, stirring constantly, for about a minute. Add the broth, and bring to a boil, reduce heat and simmer, covered, for 10 minutes or until liquid is absorbed.

Transfer pilaf to a bowl; sprinkle with cashews and scallions.

2 servings

❧

RAVIOLI WITH TOMATO AND GARLIC SAUCE

A lot of these recipes can be made even shorter and simpler. In this one, for instance, you can buy olives that are already pitted. And you don't have to worry about peeling and seeding the tomatoes—they'll be fine just chopped. The ravioli you can buy already made; all you have to do is cook it. You can even buy garlic that's already been minced. Feeling tired? Be good to yourself and take a deserved break.

1/4 cup olive oil

6 garlic cloves, minced

12 plum tomatoes, peeled, seeded, and chopped

2 pounds fresh chicken ravioli

2/3 cup chopped parsley

1/2 cup black Mediterranean olives, pitted and halved

Grated soy cheese

Heat the oil in a saucepan over medium heat. Add the garlic and cook until soft, about 3 minutes. Add the tomatoes, raise the heat to high, and cook about 10 more minutes.

Cook the ravioli. Drain. Meanwhile, reheat the garlic-and-tomato mixture if cold. Remove from heat; add the parsley and olives.

Top the ravioli with the garlic-and-tomato mixture. Serve with grated soy cheese.

4 servings

ᴁ

ORZO WITH ONION

Orzo—the pasta that looks like rice! It's slick stuff, and this is a nice little recipe.

1 garlic clove, minced
2 cups water
1 cup orzo
1 1/2 tablespoons olive oil

1 onion, chopped
1 tablespoon minced
   parsley

Bring the garlic and water to a boil in a heavy saucepan. Add the orzo and return to a boil. Reduce heat and simmer until orzo is tender, about 10 minutes. Remove from the heat and drain. Add the oil, onion, and parsley and mix well.

4 servings

ᴁ

GREEK RAINBOW TROUT

2 rainbow trout fillets
1 small tomato, chopped
1/2 cup soy cheese,
   crumbled
2 tablespoons Greek olives,
   pitted and sliced

2 teaspoons chopped
   fresh basil, or 1 tea-
   spoon dried
2 teaspoons olive oil
1/4 cup lemon juice
Lemon slices

Put the trout in a microwave dish. Sprinkle with tomato, cheese, olives, and basil. Drizzle with the olive oil and lemon juice.

Microwave on high, covered, for 2 minutes. Rotate the dish and cook 2 to 4 minutes longer on high, until fish is done. Garnish with lemon slices.

2 servings

🐟

SWORDFISH WITH GRAPEFRUIT AND ROSEMARY SAUCE

3 tablespoons margarine or butter
2 4-ounce swordfish steaks
2 shallots, minced
1 teaspoon dried rosemary, crumbled

3/4 cup fresh grapefruit juice
Fresh parsley sprigs

Melt 1 tablespoon of the margarine or butter in a heavy skillet over medium heat. Add the fish and cook until it reaches desired doneness. Transfer to a warm platter and cover to keep warm.

Add the shallots and rosemary, stirring over medium heat, until the shallots soften, about 2 minutes. Add the grapefruit juice and bring to a boil, scraping up all bits. Boil until sauce is the consistency of syrup, about 3 to 4 minutes.

Remove from the heat and add the remaining 2 tablespoons of margarine or butter, 1 tablespoon at a time, stirring until the margarine is melted. Spoon the sauce over the fish and garnish with parsley.

2 servings

&a

SCALLOPS WITH ORANGE-GINGER SAUCE

There are three kinds of sesame oil. The first is hot sesame oil, which will turn your throat into the sunward side of the planet Mercury. The second is plain, golden-colored sesame oil—it has no particular character and could be any oil. What you want is toasted sesame oil, which you can find at your local health food store. It is wonderfully flavorful stuff, and it really makes this recipe work.

3 tablespoons *fresh* orange juice (most concentrates contain added sugar)
1½ tablespoons lemon juice
1½ teaspoons grated gingerroot

1½ teaspoons cornstarch
1½ teaspoons sesame oil
¾ pound bay scallops
¾ cup cornstarch
2 tablespoons margarine or butter

In a small bowl mix orange juice, lemon juice, gingerroot, cornstarch, and sesame oil. Dip the scallops in the cornstarch mixture, coat well, and sauté in margarine or butter for 3 minutes.

Remove the scallops to a warmed serving plate. Add the orange-juice mixture to pan, raise heat to high, and reduce until thick. Pour over scallops and serve.

2 servings

❧

BROILED FISH WITH CAPER SAUCE

Trout, flounder, and sole work especially well in this recipe.

4 boneless fish fillets
    (about 1½ pounds)
4 tablespoons margarine or
    butter
2 teaspoons balsamic vin-
    egar

1½ teaspoons capers,
    rinsed
1 tablespoon minced
    parsley

Preheat the broiler. Broil the fish about 6 inches from the heat for 3 to 5 minutes.

In a small saucepan, melt the margarine or butter over low heat. Add the vinegar and capers and cook until heated through, about a minute. Remove from heat and stir in the parsley. Spoon over fillets and serve.

4 servings

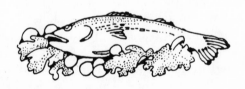

⁊

LEMON CHICKEN WITH CAPERS

This dish defines "elegant." A truly delicious, easy, and healthy recipe—we could eat something like this every night.

1/4 cup pine nuts
4 chicken breast halves,
    boned, skin on or off
1 tablespoon extra-virgin
    olive oil
1/2 cup chicken stock

1 1/2 tablespoons fresh
    lemon juice
1 tablespoon capers
3 tablespoons margarine
    or butter

Toast pine nuts in 400-degree oven or toaster oven. It won't take long, maybe 2 or 3 minutes, so keep an eye on them. Set aside to cool.

Gently pound the breasts between sheets of wax paper until flattened. In a large skillet, heat the oil over moderately high heat until almost smoking. Add breasts, skin-side down, and cook until golden brown, about 5 minutes. Turn over and cook until white throughout but still moist, an additional 3 minutes. Arrange the chicken on a large platter. Cover with foil to keep warm. Pour off fat from skillet.

Add chicken stock and bring to a boil, scraping up any brown bits from the bottom of the pan. Cook over high heat until reduced by half, about 3 minutes. Add the lemon juice and capers. Remove from heat and whisk in margarine or butter, a tablespoon at a time. Pour any accumulated juices from the chicken platter into the sauce. Pour sauce over the chicken and sprinkle with pine nuts.

4 servings

🔊

TURKEY MEAT LOAF

Our good friend Paula taste-tested this recipe and had two things to say about it: Great and easy. Or Q.E.D., as we are now saying.

2 pounds ground turkey
1½ cups fresh whole-wheat
   bread crumbs
½ cup red onion, chopped
   fine
½ cup red pepper,
   chopped fine .

1 6-ounce can tomato
   paste
2 eggs, beaten
¼ cup chopped parsley
2 teaspoons sage
4 garlic cloves, minced
1 tablespoon lemon juice

Preheat oven to 350 degrees F. Combine all ingredients in a large bowl. Mix well. Shape into loaves and place in baking pans. Bake in preheated oven for about an hour.

6 servings

🕭

TURKEY WITH GREEN PEPPERCORN SAUCE

Turkey breast slices by themselves don't have a lot of flavor—it's all in the sauce you use. This broth-onion-mustard-peppercorn one is delicious, but you can probably think of other mixtures. Olives-broth-garlic, for instance. Or one of the sauce recipes in this book—tomato, marinara...

1¼ pounds turkey breast
    slices
1 tablespoon oil
2 tablespoons margarine or
    butter
1 cup chicken broth

3 scallions, minced
1 tablespoon Dijon
    mustard
½ tablespoon green pep-
    percorns

Put turkey slices between sheets of wax paper and pound with meat-tenderizing mallet.

Heat oil and margarine or butter in a large skillet and sauté turkey slices for 2 minutes on each side. Remove and keep warm.

Simmer chicken broth, scallions, mustard, and peppercorns in the same skillet for 5 minutes. Keep heat low, or sauce will boil away. Return turkey slices to pan until warmed through, toss with sauce, and serve.

6 servings

❧

TURKEY SCALLOPS WITH CHEESE AND ARTICHOKE PURÉE

1½ tablespoon margarine
or butter
1½ tablespoon olive oil
8 turkey scallops (about
1 pound)

1 6-ounce jar marinated
artichoke hearts,
drained and puréed
4 ounces soy cheese,
grated

Heat broiler. Heat margarine or butter and olive oil in a large skillet. Add scallops; sauté until browned on both sides, about 3 to 5 minutes. Put the scallops in a large baking pan. Spread a thin layer of artichoke purée on each scallop and top with pieces of cheese.

Broil until cheese is golden and bubbly, about 4 minutes.

4 servings

❧

CURRIED LAMB WITH ORANGES

This is a great-tasting entrée, another crowd-pleaser. If you're feeling fancy, you could garnish this with orange slices. If you're tired, forget it.

1 pound lamb, trimmed of
fat and cut in 1-inch
squares
1 onion, chopped
2 garlic cloves, minced

2 teaspoons oil
1 orange, juiced
1 tablespoon curry
powder

Sauté lamb in 1 teaspoon of the oil until browned on all sides. Set aside and keep warm.

Sauté the onion and garlic in the remaining oil until the onion is tender. Add the orange juice and curry powder and stir until smooth. Cover and simmer for 8 minutes over low heat. If too dry, add more juice or a little water.

Arrange lamb on plates and cover with sauce.

6 servings

❧

ORANGE VEAL CHOPS

1/4 cup unsalted margarine or butter, softened
1/2 teaspoon grated orange rind
1 teaspoon grated lemon rind
1 teaspoon lemon juice
2 teaspoons minced shallot
1/4 teaspoon minced garlic
2 tablespoons chopped fresh basil leaves
2 tablespoons olive oil
4 1-inch-thick rib veal chops (10 ounce each)

Mix the first seven ingredients in a small mixing bowl. Chill 15 minutes. Roll into a log, wrap in wax paper, and refrigerate another hour. Make this in advance, if you wish.

In a large pan heat the oil over high heat until it is hot but not smoking. Sauté the veal chops about 10 minutes, or until meat is done to your taste, turning once.

Cut margarine or butter into half-inch slices and place on chops. Serve.

Note: Margarine or butter log can be made in advance and kept up to a month in the freezer.

4 servings

❧ Part Four ❧

Food You Don't Prepare Yourself

As we noted earlier, the world was not set up for people who need this diet. Trying to order at restaurants can be infuriating—there's not *one thing* you can eat. Delis and fast food outlets drive you crazy. The general outlook in ready-to-eat food is grim.

But it's not a total loss. We'll try to summarize here what *is* available to you.

Restaurants

You should *always* ask at restaurants about the ingredients in things. Does the tomato sauce contain sugar? Is there vinegar in anything you're ordering? Don't worry about being a pain in the neck. Make the waiter go to the kitchen and ask, if he doesn't know. Eventually you'll get a dinner you can eat.

Mexican is a good bet. You'll need to specify corn tortillas instead of flour, but the rice and beans are right on the mark. You have to be careful about cheese; request that it be left off. Especially try the El Pollo Loco fast food chain for quick, healthy, and delicious takeout.

Chinese is deadly. Almost everything has soy sauce or sugar on it. Likewise, Thai food. You can get by fairly well in a Japanese restaurant—just ask questions and read the menu carefully. Sushi, unfortunately, is a problem—the green mustard is a no-no, and raw fish may contain parasites. Parasites

183

are unfortunately all too common in people with immune-suppressed disorders, and this is one additional problem you don't need.

Middle Eastern restaurants offer falafel, which is made from vegetables. Served with tahini sauce, it's delicious. Usually they give you a salad; ask for oil and lemon juice instead of whatever other dressing they use. Hummus (made with chickpeas) is also on the approved list.

Grill restaurants are good. Grilled fish, chops, and the like are simple, delicious, and dietetically correct. Likewise, seafood restaurants. Just be sure to ask what seasonings and other ingredients are used.

At other restaurants, it's catch-as-catch-can. In some cases, the kitchen will work with you to tailor a meal to your needs. Other times this is not an option. Patience and fortitude are called for.

Takeout

As with restaurant eating, you'll probably do best with Mexican, Middle Eastern, and seafood takeout. You can even try various fried chicken places—however, fried chicken is often dipped in a wheat batter before cooking, and wheat is not allowed if you're allergic to it. Fried foods are on the forbidden list, but in an emergency (or if you're too tired to deal with anything else), you can get by with them.

Remember—ask about ingredients. Don't assume any food is okay until you know it is.

Delicatessen

There are many ready-to-eat foods you can buy at a deli or in the deli section of a supermarket. Once again, check the ingredients, and don't be surprised if this leads to the discovery that you shouldn't eat most of the foods offered.

One of our local health markets carries something called "Brown Rice Salad." It's brown rice, vegetables, and olive oil, and it is fine. The market also has tabbouleh. Other than that, there is very little.

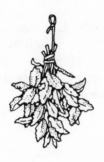

A Final Note

It has been our pleasure to put this book together for you. Eight years of our lives have been devoted to grappling with an immune system disease, and how to eat to help combat it.

Believe us when we tell you that we know the hardships and pain you face in trying to hang on to what you once thought of as your birthright: an active, healthy life. The long and winding road to rebuilding your immune system is difficult and uncertain. The medical community is still in disagreement about the best way to cope with many chronic illnesses, the insurance company won't pay your bills, and all too often you don't even have the energy to get out of bed and face the day. But our hope is that this book will help you retrieve and maintain the blessed gift of health.

With much love,

Mary and Chris

✍ Index ✍